The Complete G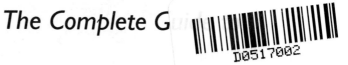

UNDERSTANDING

and

LIVING

with COPD:

From a COPDer's Perspective

R. D. Martin

Published by Every Breath, LLC, Rye Brook, NY 10573

ISBN Number: 1449946895
ISBN-13 Number: 9781449946890

Library of Congress Control Number: 2009913357

ACKNOWLEDGEMENTS

Thanks to Dusty Oliver, RRT, for inspiring me to learn as much as I can about COPD. Your halo continues to brighten many paths. Thanks also to Dr. Stuart McCalley for his tremendous help and support. Almost everything I learned about the legal aspects and paperwork involved in preparing for the inevitable, I learned from Tracy Christen Reimann, Esq. Out of my respect for her help, kindness, and sensitivity, I have suspended telling lawyer jokes until her retirement.

I am also grateful to my sister, Karen Jurgens, for her help in proofreading my book, biting her tongue when necessary, and for her well-intentioned, although unsuccessful efforts to convince me to delete immature jokes about flatulence. Thanks also to Dot Baillargeon, Mary MacDougall, Judy Wardlow, Pat Banks, Ellen Dobrin, and my other Internet friends for supporting my efforts to write this book, and tolerating my long-winded first draft.

THE COMPLETE GUIDE TO UNDERSTANDING AND LIVING WITH COPD:

FROM A COPDER'S PERSPECTIVE

By: R. D. Martin

Chapter 1

UPON BEING DIAGNOSED WITH COPD

You teach best what you most need to learn.
~ *Richard David Bach*

Having lung disease really stinks! I'm sorry you have the need to read this book. Obviously, you or someone you care about has COPD (chronic obstructive pulmonary disease). I've been dealing with it—suffering, fighting and learning about it—for close to twenty years. In addition to my own personal experience with lung disease, this book is the result of the sharing of experiences and knowledge of countless other people with COPD I've encountered over these many years who unselfishly passed on their knowledge and tips for living with COPD.

COPD is either emphysema or chronic bronchitis or both. If you have either one (or both), you have COPD. There are other lung diseases that are similar to COPD but are not technically COPD. I'll explain the medical and technical stuff later—enough to answer most of your questions. Although understanding the disease in a "clinical" sense is important, many of us find that learning about the medical details of the disease is the hardest material to read. I've taken that into consideration, so you needn't fear reading further. Although I am writing this mainly to you, the person who has COPD, people who know or work with people who have COPD will also benefit by learning about the many ways it affects our lives. If you are not the person who has COPD, but are reading this because someone you care about has COPD, you will be much better prepared to be his or her friend, proud child, loving partner, coach, sounding board, or whatever else that person needs to cope with this appalling disease. Best, when that person grits his or her teeth and curses at you out of frustration, you'll compassionately understand where he or she is coming from…a much better response than trying to find a hit man. Hit men are very pricey these days, and they get testy about being paid on time.

There is a good chance that hearing your diagnosis of COPD was very upsetting, even if you had a hunch you had COPD. Your doctor may even have been a bit of a jerk in how he or she told you that you had COPD—or failed to explain much about the disease. Unfortunately, that is all too common. There is even a chance the doctor screwed up by telling you how many years you have left to live! You may have left your doctor's office without asking the questions you now realize you "should" have asked. Once reaching the parking lot, you may have even asked yourself the ultimate question, "Why me?" as you gazed up at the heavens. If you are or were a smoker, you undoubtedly might have started to answer your own question and found your head echoing with self-incriminations, the last thing you need to hear! If COPD is new to you, you'll have plenty of time to figure out what having COPD means and what you need to do to help yourself.

Now that you've learned of your diagnosis, you have little choice but to deal with it, and deal with it you will. We all have our own ways of coping with problems, and you will find that as the challenges and problems increase, so will your coping skills. If you've been to hell and back already in your life, you probably have more coping skills at your disposal than someone who hasn't been tested as rigorously. This book is about living and coping with COPD—understanding the disease and facing the many types of problems those of us who have it encounter, such as working when you have a disability, getting the best medical care available, applying for disability, keeping your wits together, and using tricks to make your life physically easier. Heck, we'll even look way down the road so that you are prepared to make appropriate plans for your future. Of course, the problems we face are varied—widely depending on where each of us is along the path of progression of this disease and how we have adjusted to it. I'll take you on the "typical" journey of someone with COPD—from those of us still working and only beginning to struggle with illness, to those of us all too experienced with COPD.

The disease is invasive; it affects the whole of our life. Trying to deal with all the fallout it causes can leave us confused, overwhelmed, and at times even depressed. When this happens, it is always important to remember that *you are not the disease* and that you are more than just a COPD patient. You are still the spouse, parent, sibling, relative, or friend that others know and love. You have a disease; the disease does not have you.

Try your best to maintain the perspective that COPD is "influencing" your life rather than "taking over" your life. Your life will continue to be about enjoyment, making choices, accepting what you can't change, facing challenges, and adapting. There will be challenges to how you see yourself, challenges to your relationships, probably changes in your income, limitations on your mobility, and even changes to your beliefs about the meaning of life and death. Our disease teaches us quite a few hard lessons even though those lessons might, at times, feel like punishments. You may find you need to say goodbye to some of your dreams—dreams of what you imagined your future might be like before you heard you had COPD. Dreams are important—they can motivate us to move forward, and, at times, dreams are all we have to hold on to.

If we open our eyes and look around, we see healthy people with all the opportunities we could ever wish for, but if we look closely enough, we will also see that many of them are miserable. We also can't help but notice that there are people who have very little, but find many reasons to smile; some are downright happy! Having COPD does not sentence you to a life of misery any more than having good health guarantees you happiness. As we lament over our illness, we must remind ourselves that at least we're still around to complain and annoy people! Yet as much as we COPDers have in common, we are all different. You will deal with this disease in your own unique way. Fortunately, you won't need to reinvent the wheel or forge many new paths: there have been many people, far too many, who have been on this path before you who have passed on useful information. You will, nevertheless, have to endure all the bumps in the road even though I'll try to install some shock absorbers on your rear end.

Many of us need those shocks absorbers especially when we see the serious impact our health and special needs often have upon the rest of our family, especially caregivers. Not surprisingly, we find that it brings out the best and the worst from those around us, and sometimes we are even shocked by their reactions to us. Occasionally we are shocked by our own reactions! I'll help you better understand what is happening to you and your family so you can make the best of your unique situation.

Sadly and all too often, we have to fight the impact our disease has upon our emotions and mental health. We can get so distracted fighting for our physical well-being that we are depleted of energy or forget to put up a good fight to enjoy what we do have. Worse, we often have to deal with the panic of trying to catch our breath or the overwhelming sadness and depression that steals our ability to enjoy what we have. As we go on with our lives, we must cope with tremendous ongoing losses both due directly to our illness as well as to losses that are just part of living and getting older. It can feel like an assault. Further, as we try desperately to deal with our limitations, some of those around us might simply not "get it" —they don't fully understand or accept the limitations imposed upon us by our disease. Occasionally they even think we're exaggerating, or worse, they blame us and not the disease for some of the problems! We must constantly learn to keep our heads above the water and not allow the limitations of others to push us down. However, out of all the struggles and challenges, frustrations and tears, and even bouts of depression, we can still find ways to continue to grow, rejoice, and enjoy life. COPD is not a death sentence, it is a life sentence, and we'll look at how to make the best of our lives with COPD and perhaps even how to find meaning in this mess we find ourselves in.

Yes, you'll "probably" be dealing with COPD the rest of your life; I say "probably" because some of you younger readers might be around for quite a long time because of some promising breakthroughs in the treatment of COPD. There are incredible medical developments on the horizon, although we still have a few hours before the dawn. There is no doubt that we will one day be able to reverse the disease and re-grow healthy lung tissue, something currently impossible. However, taking advantage of newer treatments might buy some of us enough time to benefit until the next medical breakthrough. Even if it is a long shot, go for it; you have nothing to lose! The bottom line is that no one can predict how long you will live—a thought that has probably already entered your mind. "No one" includes your doctor. COPD progresses rapidly in some people and slowly in others. Although you have some control over the disease, when your time is up, your time is up. Hey, instead of reading this book you could be out gallivanting and get hit by a garbage truck!

Chapter 2

TELLING OTHERS OF YOUR DIAGNOSIS

What we want to tell, we wish our friend to have curiosity to hear.
~ Samuel Richardson

If you were recently diagnosed, your first impulse will probably be to share this important news with others. However, how you share your diagnosis with others is important. It is always hard to determine who is taking care of whom in such circumstances. Indeed, the person telling someone of his or her diagnosis often ends up trying to comfort the other person! When you tell others of your diagnosis, what they hear is not only dependent upon what you say, but also *how* you say it, which will be colored by your feelings at the moment. Also, what they hear will also be colored by *their* feelings and beliefs about COPD or illness in general! Telling your spouse or partner of your diagnosis usually involves much more than telling others, because your illness will probably change your partner's life almost as much as it does yours. We'll talk more about telling your partner in a later chapter.

Remember that those you tell that you have COPD will have reactions that are often very unlike your reaction. They often have images of COPD and its impact upon the future that are very different than your images. You'll have plenty of opportunities later to influence how they see you or others with COPD, so don't worry about it now. Their perceptions and beliefs, like yours, will change over time as they learn and deal with your diagnosis. It is time for you to be patient. Accept their reaction without judgment—whether their reaction pleases you or not. Save your analysis of their reaction for later. Set your expectations aside and remember *"whatever is, is."*

How you tell them might depend on who they are. Remember that most often, but not always, they will try to comfort you. You, not they, will obviously be the initial focus. Oddly enough, there is often a turnaround, and you will be in the position, without even realizing it, of reassuring them! You might walk away feeling worse because of their distress and feel compelled to "take care" of their feelings. Be loving, kind, and considerate, but remember that you are not the cause of their distress; the illness is! They may walk away feeling "ill-prepared" to deal with you, COPD, or the future; that is not unusual. Therefore, keep your conversation focused on the present. If fears about the future come up during the conversation, as they often do, explain that there will be plenty of time to prepare for the future. You can reassure both of you with the reminder that you will figure out how to handle things in the future.

Be aware that there might be great awkwardness when you tell them of your diagnosis; you'll both perhaps feel uncomfortable. You might even feel more like an actor than yourself. If so, that's okay. Your health, or more correctly how healthy you "appear," has a lot to do with how they might react. We COPDers can look pretty darn healthy! Often, when told of your COPD, they will attempt to reach out and find common ground even though what they say might not be the most suitable comment. At other times, they try to immediately relate it to their own experience and consequently make some seemingly insensitive statements. Here are some possibilities:

1. "Oh, a lot of people are told they have COPD (or emphysema) and they get along just fine. I wouldn't worry about it if I were you."

2. "Your chances of getting hit by a car are greater than the chance that you will die of it. Why, just the other day a thirty-seven-year-old marathon runner dropped dead..."

3. "What else did the doctor say? Other than that, how are you doing?"

4. "Oh, my grandmother had that," and...blah, blah, blah about granny.

5. "How long does the doctor think you have?"

6. "Join the club, I have gout, arthritis, a heart murmur and..."

7. "It is probably nothing; those doctors always come up with things to scare you."

8. "From smoking?"

9. "So, what are you going to do?"

10. "Oh, my God, I can't believe it!"

11. "You should sue those damn tobacco companies. They..."

12. "Are you going to get a lung transplant?"

13. "You will be in all of my prayers."

14. "Well, remember, that's just one doctor's opinion. You should always get a second opinion. Did you ask him..."

15. "So, who's going to take care of you?"

16. "When you die, can I have your car?"

17. "Gee, I don't know what to say!"

18. "Well, you're going to have to start taking better care of yourself!"

19. "Don't worry about it. We're all going out one way or another."

20. "Don't worry; everything is in God's hands."

Let's take a look at some of the above, because they fall into common categories. Knowing this, you'll be better prepared to respond to others' reactions.

Seven Reactions of Others to Being Told You Have COPD

1. **Minimizing:** People who minimize the news because they can't deal with the importance or significance of it. Either they don't really understand it or can't deal with the emotional impact it might have upon them or you—at least not at that moment. This does not mean that they don't care about you. They usually need more time to let it sink in.

2. **Overreacting:** God bless these caring people, and, yes, you'll have to reassure them that, with their help, you'll make the best of it. Although it can be scary if people overreact (if you start wondering if you are under reacting), let them know how much they mean to you and how important their support is. In time, they'll hook into your "can do" attitude, and there is a good chance that they will be there for you in the long run.

3. **Zeroing In:** Some people will "zero in" to immediately gather all the information they can, as if they are handling an emergency hotline. This is annoying because they are usually moving faster

than you. You do not have to be pulled in their direction or go at their speed. Simply let them know that there is plenty of time to gather all the information they are worried about. These people find that questions and answers are easier to deal with than raw feelings.

4. **Selfish Reaction**: Some people, unfortunately, will immediately think only of about how your illness will impact them. Yup, they are asses. You are free to say anything you want to them and amend your will accordingly.

5. **Speechless:** Some people are just going to be speechless or run at the mouth (but say little that is meaningful), be awkward, stumble, be silent, or even say that they don't know what to say. These are good people, and they are dealing with it emotionally—or at least trying to. If they are not equipped to say the right thing at the right time, so be it. You can take the pressure off of them and let them know that it is awkward for you, too, and that there will be plenty of time to talk in the future. Let them know that you care about them. Don't judge their awkwardness. Awkwardness is not a bad sign.

6. **Anger:** Yup, some people will react to your news with anger— anger at the tobacco companies, at the government for allowing the sale of poisons, at you for smoking, etc! Although low on the list of reactions you would like to have, bottom line is that they are angry that you are injured. That is not necessarily a bad thing; however, don't spend a lot of time with them or add fuel to their anger. Anger, be it yours or theirs, can perhaps one day be channeled into putting up a good fight, but for the time being, it might get in the way.

7. **I'm Here for You**: Some people just have the right words to say and will manage to convey their deep concern for you, keep the focus on you, and offer current and future support. Some people immediately say the right words, and some may stammer before coming up with the right words. God bless these people!

Watch Body Language

Remember to observe others' body language and not just listen with your ears. Do they cross their arms as if to protect themselves from your news? Do they slouch or rest their head upon their hands because of the heavy mental burden? Do they hold your hand, put their hand on your shoulder, or even hug you to physically connect with you? Sometimes the words will match the body language and sometimes not. Trust the body language before you trust the words.

Remember That Your Diagnosis Affects Everyone

If you are part of a family, your health and needs affect or will eventually affect everyone. Your diagnosis is not just a personal problem, it is a family problem, and the reaction you get from some people might reflect that. Some families and some individuals within the family are better able to deal with your news than others. What is wonderful and perhaps surprising, and new territory for a few of us, is that you have some control over how family members deal with your diagnosis and your illness. Eventually, having COPD often puts a strain on relationships. It has the potential to turn lovers and spouses into caregivers, children into nurturers and caregivers, turn siblings against each other, and scare some people off. For others of us who do not even have families with whom to share this diagnosis, it is perhaps even worse. COPD is not just about your lungs; it is about your life in all its complexity and all its meaning. For most of us, it is the greatest challenge of our lives. Keep in mind not only for yourself, but when you share your diagnosis with others, that having COPD does not signal the end of your life. It is only the beginning of a new phase of life.

When you tell people you have COPD, a large number will ask if you were a smoker. If you were or are a smoker, you may be very uncomfortable with this question. Harder than answering them, you have to answer to yourself, and you must face the reality that you caused or contributed to your disease. If you are a smoker or former smoker, you probably need help to reconcile the past with the present and to deal with this oppressive ghost straightaway.

Chapter 3

FOR YOU SMOKERS AND FORMER SMOKERS

But they whose guilt within their bosoms lie imagine every eye behold their blame.
~William Shakespeare

One of the first things that many people think of when they hear about COPD (chronic obstructive pulmonary disease) is smoking. If you were a smoker (or still are), either you are going to blame yourself for your condition, or others will inevitably blame you. Even if they don't, you will probably imagine (according to Shakespeare) that they are blaming you, so it is all the same anyway! First, not all COPD is caused by smoking. If you use the word "emphysema" with people (remember that emphysema and chronic bronchitis are the two types of COPD, and that you can have both), they are more likely to associate it with smoking. If you use the acronym COPD, they might be less familiar with the meaning and therefore a bit less likely to ask that dreaded question. You might want to use both terms depending on your mood and who asks. Now, we all know that if someone asks the question about smoking, most expect to hear that you were a smoker. We also know that they are probably predisposed to holding you accountable for your illness, putting you down, or making you feel uncomfortable. The exception is doctors; smoking history is actually important information for them. Because many people, outside of doctors, want to make you admit it out loud, you are therefore entitled to have some fun with them. Here are some possible responses to the question of smoking:

Have Some Fun with Them
- Yes, I did smoke. I have smoked since I was seven years old. My daddy worked for a tobacco company, and as children we were made to chain-smoke in case his boss dropped by. Come to think of it, he never did drop by!

- No, it must have been caused by secondhand smoke. (By the way, this may be true for some of you, so I apologize for putting it here.)

- I have the inherited type. (This, too, is true for some people, and I again apologize. *Mea culpa, mea culpa!*)

- Hell yes, like a damn chimney, I tell you! I enjoyed every one. Got one you can spare? From the looks of your complexion, I can tell you're a smoker!

- Smoking kept my mental illness under control. Whenever I stop, I start having homicidal thoughts. As a matter of fact, I stopped again recently and those terrible thoughts are returning. You are not Satan, are you?

- Yes, I got COPD from smoking and now encourage everyone I know to stop smoking. If you invite me over for dinner, I'll come over and scare the hell out of your kids. Are you a halfway decent cook? I certainly hope so. I usually eat about 6:00, is that too early for you?

- No, I didn't smoke—well, except for crack cocaine when I wasn't incarcerated.

Bottom line is that you should not let them succeed in trying to make you feel guilty or bad. Although easier said than done, it is within in your control. People can't make you feel bad, guilty, or anything else. All they can do is push your button—you know, that guilt button in your head labeled "*guilt.*" They know it is there, so put some electrical tape over that button!

The smoking that caused or contributed to your lung disease is in the past. You can't change the past, regardless of how often your mind goes there. I find it interesting that people consider it acceptable to ask about smoking when you have COPD. Would you ask them if they were a lousy driver if they told you they were in a car accident? Certainly, being a lousy driver contributes to the probability of having an accident as much as smoking contributes to COPD! If they get colon cancer, do you ask them if they ate the recommended amount of roughage? If they get diabetes, do you ask if they were too fond of sweets, or, if they had a heart attack, if they ate the proper diet and got enough exercise? Feel free to share these observations with them—just be aware that you might not see them again.

You can forgive yourself in the same manner you forgive others for their imperfections or past actions. If you are a rather unforgiving person, it will be harder for you. Forgiveness is stressed in many religious and belief systems. You can apologize to yourself if you feel that is beneficial. Another way is to simply catch yourself when you think about your role in the formation of your disease and put an abrupt end to the mind chatter. If you start thinking guilty thoughts, simply stop and think of something else, something more pleasant. If you practice this, after enough repetition, you will find that you change the chatter, and in doing so you let go of much of the guilt. Guilt ceases to exist if it has no voice, and not thinking about something can be a way of letting go of it. At first, you'll be surprised how frequently those negative thoughts arise. It takes quite a bit of repetition, so stick with it. This is not to say that you won't be reminded of your past actions when you see someone run when you can't, or dance when all you can do it tap your foot, but your regrets will be more manageable if they are not accompanied by unnecessary guilt. I just tell myself, for example, that this illness happened for a reason, and although I don't understand why, I'm not expected to figure it out. It works for me.

Now that you are beginning to deal with your diagnosis and thinking about the future and the impact the disease will possibly have on your life, it is important to understand what COPD is, and equally important to dispel some myths about COPD by also looking at what COPD is not! Although reading about a disease is difficult and far from pleasant reading, not understanding your disease will probably be even more difficult, so it is best to forge ahead. It is not as scary as you might think.

Chapter 4

COPD: WHAT IT IS AND WHAT IT IS NOT

The more serious the illness, the more important it is for you to fight back, mobilizing all your resources—spiritual, emotional, intellectual, and physical.
~ *Norman Cousins*

COPD stand for Chronic, Obstructive, Pulmonary Disease. It is a very serious disease, and like most serious diseases, it permeates every aspect of our lives, sometimes even our dreams at night. I no longer walk stairs in my dreams and even explain to those with the nerve to appear in my dreams that "I don't do stairs."

COPD Affects a Large Number of People
COPD is an enormous problem. The numbers are astronomical: it claims between 100,000 and 200,000 Americans each year. Between 80% and 90% of COPD is caused by smoking (there are other causes). Over 11 million or 12 million people in the United States have it, and another 24 million have evidence of reduced lung function or have it and have not been formally diagnosed. One more scary figure I've read is that it is (when combined with asthma) the leading cause of death in the United States for those of us over forty-five years old! When not combined with asthma, it is often cited as the fourth leading cause of death in the United States, and one in four families has a member with COPD. Obviously, the numbers are staggering, and this means that you are not alone; however there is only one person with COPD that matters right now, and that is you. Just because a lot of people have it doesn't make it a bit easier for you.

What COPD Is
COPD is lung damage that, by definition, is chronic (always present or reoccurring), obstructs (blocks or hinders) the movement of air *out* of the lungs, and "pulmonary" (which simply means related to the lungs). By the way, if something interferes with air going *into* the lungs, it is called a "restrictive" disease instead of an "obstructive" disease.

However, many of us with COPD have a lesser restrictive component to our COPD anyway, so we have both. The term COPD usually only refers to chronic bronchitis and emphysema, but you'll occasionally see "asthma" thrown in, too, because there are often asthmatic components to chronic bronchitis and emphysema. Further, a few medical people include bronchiectasis (a disease that causes dilation of the bronchial tree) into the category of COPD. There are, of course, other obstructive and restrictive lung diseases, but I'm sticking to the topic of COPD. Nevertheless, the consequences of not breathing well and the ways in which people with other lung diseases cope with the limitations may be similar regardless of diagnosis.

How the Lungs Work

I will give you a brief overview of how the lungs work, because that is all the information that is necessary. There is more than enough information readily available for those who want more clinical information about the physical manifestation of the disease.

We depend on oxygen (O2) to live. The air we normally breathe contains about 21% O2 at sea level plus other gasses such as nitrogen, argon, and a tad (less than 1%) of carbon dioxide (CO2). Our lungs absorb O2 from air to fuel our body, including all of our organs. Carbon dioxide (CO2) is the end product that our bodies produce after we break down nutrition. We exhale that CO2. Simply put, our lungs extract O2 from the air and use it for our metabolism, which produces CO2 as a byproduct, like fumes from an engine. We then discharge the CO2 when we breathe out. We need the right balance of both CO2 and O2 in our bodies to remain healthy. Breathing is, therefore, not just about getting enough O2; it is equally about getting rid of enough CO2.

Our lungs, two of them, are not like the large balloons that many people imagine. Instead, they are a series of hollow branches (think of a hollow tree) called bronchial tubes. Off of these branches are little air sacs that are designed to exchange O2 and CO2 (think of these as plump leaves on the branches). These little sacs are called "alveoli" and are bunched together. "Alveoli" is one of only a few fancy medical terms I'll use, so be patient. The proper exchange of gasses is also related to keeping our body's pH (acid/alkaline) level where it should be, a vitally important function. COPD is a disease that destroys the lung tissue we need in order for our lungs to carry this necessary exchange of gasses. This exchange, by the way, is called "diffusion." Okay, so I snuck another medical term in! Finally, the lungs expand and contract due to the pull and release of our diaphragm. Our diaphragm is below our lungs and is a sheet of muscle used to inflate and deflate the lungs. Excuse me for the comparison, but the closest thing I can think of is a toilet plunger pushing up or down and pulling or pushing the water under it. There are also some other muscles that assist breathing. We'll get back to this later—when your headache subsides.

Anyway, COPD affects this process. Once again, there are two types of COPD (according to most definitions); however, many if not most people have at least some of both:

Chronic Bronchitis

Chronic bronchitis is ongoing inflammation of the bronchial tubes. The inflammation itself makes breathing difficult because it narrows or closes the tubes carrying the O_2 in and CO_2 out. To make matters worse, the inflammation scars the tubes, and phlegm or mucus develops. The scarring ends up thickening the tubes. This is yet another level of problems that occur because the thickening further impairs our breathing. Finally, these changes create a Disneyland for bacteria and viruses. The problem is that this Disneyland doesn't close each night for cleaning. Keeping the phlegm loose so it can slowly work its way up and you can cough it out helps the cleaning process.

Emphysema

Remember when I explained that there are little sacs off the branches in the lungs, and I annoyed you by calling them "alveoli"? Well, emphysema is the slow destruction of these alveoli so that they cannot do their job exchanging the gasses O_2 and CO_2. The destruction results in holes or spaces in the lungs. In addition, the lungs lose their elasticity, further impairing the ability of the lungs to work properly. The body compensates by trying to expand the lungs by making more room and pushing what it can aside. The diaphragm can become misshapen, and the lungs can push out on the rib cage, creating a characteristic barrel chest.

Both chronic bronchitis and Emphysema can have asthmatic components. Our airways can become inflamed or constricted—something you've probably learned from TV commercials touting the latest medications!

Causes of COPD

Most COPD is caused by smoking—probably 80% to 90%. Secondhand smoke can also cause COPD, as can exposure to other toxic substances. Marijuana smoking is especially hard on the lungs. There is research currently being done that looks at COPD as a type of autoimmune disease. Other researchers claim that genetics play a role in determining which smokers get it and which don't. I come from a family of smokers. I lost a brother to COPD, my sister has it, and my mother recently died at 98 of it. She never smoked but was around a lot of secondhand smoke.

There is also a form of emphysema that is inherited. It accounts for about 3% of people with emphysema (or 100,000 in the United States). In the inherited type, also call genetic emphysema, individuals are born with a deficiency in their ability to produce Alpha-1 Antitrypsin (AAT). This is a chemical that protects the lungs. The doctor treating you should have tested you for this as part of their initial evaluation or at least ask if you've been tested for this. It is a simple blood test, and the doctor might have tested you without even telling you, so double check to be sure this was completed. There are special medications to help you if you have the inherited type of emphysema.

The role of air pollution is still a bit unknown. At best, it probably contributes to COPD and can certainly make our breathing more difficult once we have COPD. Other indoor as well as outdoor and manufacturing pollutions may also damage the lungs. Some pollutants, such as asbestos, can lead to specific diseases that do not fall under the label of COPD.

Although asthma, or airway hyper-responsiveness, and COPD are usually considered different diseases, recent studies suggest that having asthma makes one more vulnerable than average to developing COPD later if the asthmatic smokes. In fact, many COPD patients have an "asthmatic component" to their disease—the characteristic wheezing.

What COPD Is Not

- COPD is not, to date, reversible. One day it will be, and that's a darn good reason to hang in there!

- COPD is not contagious.

- COPD is not necessarily a death sentence, although there is a good chance that it will eventually kill you directly or indirectly.

- COPD is usually not a disease that progresses rapidly. The average person has a good number of years ahead of him or her if diagnosed at the onset.

- COPD is not the end of your life or the good times.

- COPD is not something over which we have as much control as we'd like, although there are some things related to the disease that we can control.

- COPD does not decrease your ability to appreciate many of the things that life has to offer, even though it may limit you to fewer things.

COPD is not the type of damage to the lungs that we think of when we think of damage due to an injury. COPD is progressive, which is to say, the lungs continue to deteriorate over time. For this reason, it is a very difficult disease to which to adjust. As soon as we adjust to our current abilities (or is that disabilities?), those abilities become even less, and we start once again readjusting. Understanding the progression of the disease will help us prepare for the future and help us deal with the obstacles we will face. We all want to know what to expect.

Chapter 5

COPD: ITS PROGRESSION AND STAGES

Nothing is predestined: the obstacles of your past can become the gateways that lead to new beginnings.
~Anonymous

COPD is often like a very long roller coaster that starts at the summit and proceeds downhill, not always in a gradual or predictable manner, but in a manner that is erratic because of its many frightening curves and numerous ups and downs. It is also like taking this ride blindfolded, unable to see or plan for the dips and crests; it leaves you clutching for stability, always wondering when the ride will end, and convinced at times that the end is just around the next curve. Although this has been my experience, I do know a few people whose decline has been slow, gradual, and remarkably uneventful—without the dramatic ups and downs that I associate with COPD. I've also known a few people whose doctors have told them that they have mild emphysema and if they stop smoking it will not get worse. I don't buy that prognosis, although I do know a few people who seem to reach a point and remain there year after year with no discernable decline. There is tremendous variability between individuals.

The Gradual Progression Approach to Understanding COPD
In one sense, the "progression" of the disease is a simple concept: it is the continuing decline in your ability to breathe, which gradually results in you being physically able to do less. You will also experience greater SOB (shortness of breath) over time. In the beginning, physical demands upon you are minor, almost inconveniences. You can still mow your lawn, but you need to stop to catch your breath a bit more often. You can live with that. Perhaps you'll stop a bit more frequently when walking or need to sit and rest more often than before. You might find that as it becomes harder to exert yourself, you cut corners and get less exercise. Getting less exercise, I must warn you, can begin a downward spiral. Eventually, others will notice your SOB and ask if you are okay—first family and friends, and eventually maybe even

strangers. You will probably try to hide your SOB from them. Perhaps you even try to hide it from yourself, rationalizing it away—you're out of shape, getting old, etc. Before long, you are ordering a riding mower from Sears, and eventually you will even give up the riding mower because the fumes bother your breathing. Things that you never thought of as requiring energy become more difficult and become chores rather than routines. As each year passes, you are able to do less because you get out of breath more easily. The flu, colds, and respiratory infections that were just inconvenient earlier in your life become incapacitating and perhaps even life threatening. The progression of COPD is sometimes gradual and subtle. At other times, there is a noticeable step down, like descending a staircase one step (thump) at a time (usually after an illness). However, every once in a while, you might regain just a bit of what you lost and actually go back up a stair or two, sort of a reverse of the old saying "two steps forwards, one step backward." During those better times, your spirits will lift and you will remember these unexpected gifts to keep you going during the bad periods. Eventually, however, if you manage to evade your departure from this earth due to secondary or other unrelated illness, you might need help with even the simplest chores, such as walking, dressing, or bathing. At that point, many find a wheelchair or scooter the easiest way of getting around. When you begin to think of reaching this point in your life, you might be frightened and concerned about who will take care of you. This is normal and reasonable.

All too often, our hearts give out or other medical problems related to our COPD bring our life to an end before we have to deal with needing wheelchairs or becoming completely dependent. As a final kick in the pants, we may end up leaving this earth for reasons having nothing to do with COPD. There is nothing stopping you from having other medical problems, and it seems that most of us do. Always wear clean underwear just in case, and remember, if you label your underwear with the days of the week, you can always drop your pants to find out what day it is.

You will also find that as your COPD progresses, your breathing reacts negatively to many more things, such as perfumes, odorizers, smoke, any type of cleaning or chemical fumes, and even candles and cooking smells. Most of us are also negatively affected by extremes or changes in weather. High humidity, changes in barometric pressure, weather fronts, and dew points are all cited as possible causes for "bad breathing days." Yet for reasons unknown, and in spite of our predictions based on current weather conditions, we can have mysterious "good breathing days." Most of us COPDers also find that the quality of our breathing is not only about the atmosphere around us, it also has to do with our emotional state—more than we'd like to admit. Anxiety can make our breathing more difficult. Frankly, trying to understand all the possible causes can tire one out. No matter what theories you come up with, you will have days that prove your theories wrong. It is easier to accept each day as it is and give our thanks for still being around to complain about the weather.

Because of the continued loss of breathing ability as the disease progresses, your body tries to compensate, and greater stress is put on your heart and circulatory system. You therefore have an increased possibility of developing cardiac problems or other secondary illnesses. Your inability to move, exercise, and burn calories might also affect your overall health or cause yet other health problems. There is no doubt about it: having COPD is a real test and you are being tested… really, really being tested! There might be days when you wonder if the fight is worth it, so you must make your mind up now to refuse to let COPD destroy your spirit. It doesn't have to unless you let it.

Looking at COPD as Stages

Another way of looking at the progression of our disease is to put the progression into stages, which is nothing more than breaking the progression of our disease into distinct parts, sections, or phases. We love breaking things down into stages. We have a stage for everything, so there is no reason that COPD should not also have its own stages!

Medical personnel usually view or, more accurately, refer to our illness as progressing in stages. Using the concept of us going through stages is important to those who treat us. Using stages helps communicate a cluster of information in a concise format from one professional to another or to an insurance company, for example. Some doctors share with their patient the name of the stage they are in. For example, still somewhat popular but finally fading out (thankfully) is the use of the terms "mild," "moderate," "severe," and "end stage" COPD. The stages are determined primarily by pulmonary function test scores. According to this rather outdated classification, a one-point difference in the test result one way or another could be the difference between being "severe" and being "end stage." Although the differences in the scores might not be statistically significant, the emotional impact of the label is. People can go home and announce they are "end stage" and find themselves repeating their dire diagnosis and prognosis for years, scaring themselves and shortchanging themselves when it comes to receiving gifts. Be aware that people limit themselves to buying only certain types of gifts if they think they are giving it to a person who isn't going to last long. Forget jewelry or a GPS system—you won't be getting any if you tell people you are "end stage." You'll be unwrapping pajamas, slippers, and sweaters for the rest of your life!

I know people who have been diagnosed "end stage" for close to twenty years. They are not unlike aging singers who go on for decades giving final farewell performances. Some people's COPD progresses rapidly and others, very slowly. Some people even seem to come to a standstill and remain much the same year after year! To make the "stage" approach even less meaningful for the patient (I'm still not saying it doesn't have its place within professional practices), not all doctors or labs translate the test score into the same stage name. Although the raw test score numbers should be consistent between labs, the labs may use different scoring charts or scales and therefore put you into different stages. Further, people with the same scores and in the same stages might have very different physical abilities and lifestyles. Thinking in terms of stages, at least for those of us with COPD, therefore has some serious limitations.

Protesting against the overuse of placing us in stages aside, doctors are increasingly moving away from using descriptive words for stages (such as "serious" and "end stage") and have adopted numbers instead. It is a good move and might reshape attitudes, but a rose by any other name… Unfortunately, numbers (if someone is going to use a number to represent a stage) are not neutral either; they have their own associations! As an example, stage 3 in cancer carries a lot of meaning—so to be in stage 3 is absolutely not neutral! The American Thoracic Society (ATS) now recommends that physicians adopt the association's new names and criteria for stages. The stages are determined by PFTs (pulmonary function tests). The descriptions for stages below are based upon the outcomes of one of the tests, called the FEV1 (although other criteria might also be used). The FEV1 stands for forced expiratory (breathing out) volume in one second, and it is numerical score for how much air we can force out of our lungs in one second.

- **Stage 1** = 50% or more of predicted value (this is based on gender and height) for someone with normal lungs. Although one might be complaining of severe breathlessness, the overall impact upon one's life is considered minimal and can usually be treated with bronchodilators (inhalers) and/or other medications that address the inflammation or constriction. We'll explore the different medications later. This stage corresponds to the "mild" description that is falling out of use. Frankly, it doesn't feel mild when you are there!

- **Stage 2** = 35% to 49% of predicted value. At this point, there is "significant" impact upon the person's life. Inhaled corticosteroids are often added if they seem to work. These are not the anabolic steroids used in body building, but another type of steroid that is an anti-inflammatory. This corresponds to the descriptive term "moderate."

- **Stage 3** = 35% or less of predicted value. This is considered "severe" and has a profound impact upon the person's life. The whole arsenal of medications is considered if necessary, along with O2 at some point.

- Note that there is no number 4 or end stage! Thank you, American Thoracic Society!

I think you'll agree that it is just as easy to simply give the real FEV1 number or percentage of one's lung capacity because there is a wide range assigned to each stage. Most of us, I think, would prefer to hear our percentage of FEV1 than the stage. If you are given a stage name or stage number, ask for your FEV1 percentage. To be fair, it is not a conspiracy by physicians to present information in this manner. Patients often want to hear terms familiar to them such as "mild" and "severe." It takes two to tango. Frankly, there is no way to use words or numbers to make any stage of our disease sound okay. Bless them for trying, but the goal is unachievable.

The End Stage of COPD

The term "end stage" is still used by some doctors, and in fact many of us will reach our end due to COPD or its complications—whether or not we want to call it a stage! The classification "end stage" has fallen out of favor because it is not only discouraging, it also fails to live up to its name! The problem is that some people are diagnosed as being "end stage" but continue to live and enjoy life for many, many years. Telling people that they are "end stage" is not unlike blindfolding them and instructing them to walk forward while informing them that there is a cliff in front of them and it may be close or far away! Each step ahead can be terrifying, and it makes it hard to enjoy the walk. I see "end stage" as meaning that we've driven our doctors to the "end stage" of their wits trying to think of things to help us when we've exhausted their arsenal of things that could help us!

How Long Do I Have?

Many people want to know how many years they have to live. This is similar to thinking about "end stage." Although this is a very reasonable request and important information, no one really knows—really! I know someone with COPD that was given three years to live. That was fourteen years ago. Another person I know was given one year and lived twenty. The opposite can be true, too. Things happen. We've all been issued boarding passes. Have your boarding passes ready if you must, but enjoy your time here in this friendly terminal as best you can.

Meanwhile, and long before many of us have to start worrying about reaching the boarding gate, we have to keep our current lives together, which for many of us means we need to continue working! One of the most difficult challenges we have is to manage being an employee and income earner as we struggle to breathe. If you work outside of the home, you need to look ahead to ensure that you can maintain your employment as long as possible. Managing your illness while holding down a job can be very difficult, and there is a good chance you'll need all the help you can get. Fortunately, there is some help to be had!

Chapter 6

WORKING WHEN YOU HAVE COPD

Always be smarter than the people who hire you.
~*Lena Horne*

If you are working and have lung disease, you are probably finding it more and more difficult to continue working. If this hasn't happened to you yet, there is a good chance that it will when your COPD has progressed. Not only do you have your own expectations regarding what you "should" be able to do, you are no doubt struggling to balance your personal health needs with your need and desire to be a good worker and a valued employee. Perhaps you've even given up on being valued and just want to be safe and secure!

Much of our identity is often tied into our jobs. Sometimes, much of our social life is centered around people we know through our jobs, and they become as important as family members. If that isn't enough, it obviously provides us with the income we need to keep our lives going and the health insurance that we need now more than ever. Although we complain about work and even have days when we wished we didn't have to work any longer, we tend to hold on to our jobs as long as we can. In many ways, how we are handling our jobs becomes our measure of how well we are handling our illness— and our lives!

There is often a point in time when either you or your employer simply can't take it any longer—you are calling in sick too often and your work suffers tremendously. It can sometimes become painfully obvious to everyone around you before anyone says something out loud or someone takes action to deal with the problem. You may experience people distancing themselves from you in preparation for your eventual departure. Being in this situation is a terrible feeling, a feeling of really being trapped. We often begin faking the appearance of being healthier than we are and learn to wait until no one is watching before we stop to catch our breaths. We may even use our ability to work as evidence to convince ourselves that we aren't going downhill. We try to fool ourselves, but the day comes when we admit, "I can't do it any longer."

The average work situation is often stressful even for healthy people. When you add your illness into the equation, you might have a mess on your hands. Frankly, whether or not it is fair, your illness, if it is advanced, is probably affecting others at work. It is not your fault even though you probably think that it is. You might feel bad about it, even to the point of feeling guilty or depressed. It is hard not to blame yourself when those around you do. It is neither your fault nor the fault of those with whom you work. Your co-workers didn't ask for this mess anymore than you did.

You will probably want to hang on to your job as long as you can but not so long as to cause more damage to yourself in the process. There might also be the chance that your decline is related to your job environment, specifically the type of work you do, which may entail exposure to extreme weather, poor air quality at your workplace, or stress.

Sick Buildings and Air Quality at Work
There are a number of jobs that are simply more difficult to perform than others because of our COPD. There are also a number of jobs that contribute to the decline in our health because of the poor indoor or even outdoor air quality. Sometimes the poor air quality is due to work environments where there is some form of production occurring, such as manufacturing, printing, or any industry that involves fumes. In addition to these more obvious air quality issues that lead to respiratory problems, sometimes the problem is less obvious and is often due to a poor ventilation system or poorly maintained ventilation system. This is referred to as a "sick building syndrome." This disorder can occur either in select areas of a building or throughout the whole building. The "sick building syndrome" is often found in large buildings that were constructed to be heat and air-conditioning efficient. They include hospitals, schools, and office buildings. If you think that air quality is a problem, the Occupational Safety and Health Administration (OSHA) oversees work environments and is dedicated to ensuring a safe work environment. Call OSHA at 1-866-4-USA-DOL or visit www.osha.gov to find out how you should address any air quality problem at work.

Find the Best Medical Help

While you are still working, get the best medical help you can find, and do it as soon as you can. The right medical evaluation and treatment of your COPD will keep you working longer and feeling better about working.

Disability and Social Security Disability Income

The day will probably come when you are unable to work any longer, and it is a problem if you are below retirement age. You will need income, and when and if you qualify due to your COPD, you will eventually receive Social Security Disability Income (SSDI). Be aware that just being diagnosed with COPD is not enough. Your breathing has to be significantly impaired enough for you to qualify—impaired to the point where you cannot work doing *any* job, not just your current one. Applications for SSDI can be completed online or through your local Social Security office. The application process is comprehensive when it comes to ascertaining your medical conditions(s) and treatment history.

If you apply for SSDI, the staff at Social Security will review your application and collect pertinent medical records concerning your COPD. Once they have the medical information they need, either from your medical records or examinations by their own physicians, they will see if your condition meets their strict criteria. To do this, they turn to what for them is their bible—their book of medical eligibility criteria. You have to meet or surpass their criteria to qualify for SSDI. This book of criteria is referred to as the "Blue Book." By looking at their Blue Book before you apply, you are able to see what they will be looking at to determine whether you are eligible. To some extent (but only to some extent) you can find out if you have "passing" breathing test scores and/or meet other very specific criteria. Be warned that you will not be able to predict if you quality for SSDI with 100% accuracy. When you have multiple medical conditions, Social Security staff members try their best to look at the big picture. The Blue Book is available through Social Security's Web site (www.socialsecurity.gov). Currently, the page that covers respiratory illnesses is at www.ssa.gov/disability/professionals/bluebook/3.00-Respiratory-Adult.htm. If turned down, you can appeal a number of times; however, it may be a very lengthy process!

Disability (SSDI) aside, only you know how far you can push your-self. I have never been anything less than amazed at the differences in physical abilities between people with COPD. If you start looking at your test numbers and compare your results with others, you'll go nuts. Some people with the same test results (at least the numbers we tend to focus on) can be close to being bedridden, while others manage to work each day. Go figure!

I'm sure you've noticed that many people have a slight problem with sick people—they either don't seem to like them or they feel uncomfortable around them. Illness is often perceived as weakness. If you belong to a nomadic tribal group and you are sick, and it is time to take down the tents and move, your illness really is a hardship for the group—that's obvious. Similarly, if you are currently part of a team working on a cooperative project, you can become a weak link. You will not be making your co-workers happy. It is not just about them being "nice" or "understanding" about your limitations; your health can really negatively affect them. If you are in this situation, you need information and resources to help you keep the show going until you are ready to draw the curtain. In addition to your charming personality and problem-solving abilities, you might have some formal legal protections, protections available to you if you are a disabled individual.

Your Protections If You Are Working

Before we proceed, however, get down on your knees (if still possible) and kiss the ground. Express your thanks for being not only an American but for being born in an age when we have these protections. It you can't get back up off your knees, you might want to consider wearing an emergency alarm system to call for help!

If you have documented COPD, you *might* be considered to have a "disability." The impairment due to COPD, however, has to be significant. Frankly, having a mild or even moderate impairment due to COPD might not earn you formal protections simply because of the diagnosis alone. Unlike some other disabilities, your COPD probably doesn't show unless you have to stop to catch your breath, but even then some people simply don't notice it, and some of those who do notice it don't seem to "get it." Fortunately, and it's a good reason to celebrate, we have laws to protect employers from discriminating against people with disabilities, including those of us with significant breathing difficulties. If you are disabled, you have special legal protections.

When it comes to protections for people with disabilities or handicaps, as a general rule, whichever law is the most stringent is the most important. There are federal laws, state laws, and even sometimes some local laws that protect the rights of people with disabilities. We'll look at federal laws, but you might also explore state and local laws that protect you. Contact your state's Department of Labor to find all laws and regulations that apply to your workplace, and contact your county government to learn about any local laws that can protect you.

Employers generally do not like these protective laws as they require responsibility and accountability from the company and sometimes leave the organization vulnerable should its practices ever violate the protective regulations. This is not to say that employers don't believe in them; it is just that the laws require employers, at times, to make adaptations in their work environment that may include changes to their physical environment or changes in their practices, standards, policies, and staff training. Surprisingly, some companies operate rather obliviously to protective regulations; they tend to be smaller companies who do not employ professional human resource managers.

Generally speaking, the people in your organization will not protect you; the laws will. Because of the complexity of these laws and the inability of companies to train all supervisors in the applicable laws, once you declare your rights as a disabled person, you might have to interact directly with the personnel or human resources department instead of your supervisor. If you belong to a union, your union may represent you during any serious discussion and may have other recommendations or requirements that should supersede anything covered in this chapter.

Rules are rules, but your attitude is very important also. It is easy for company representatives to get a bit self-protective and even paranoid because of the consequences of not following the rules. They may also have had encounters with employees who have tried to "play the system." If you pick up on a bit of attitude, don't let it ruffle your feathers. For this reason and regardless of the rule, be it federal, state, or local, remember that the rules exist to articulate expectations for *both* you and your employer. The rules are not just about what *your company* must do, it is equally about what *you* must do. If you do not follow the rules, the rules will not be able to help you. Both employee and employer must cross all of their "t's" and dot all of their "i's." If anyone fails, one party can use it against the other. Unless absolutely impossible, keep the fear and paranoia to an absolute minimum. This requires you to be nonthreatening. Be knowledgeable and assertive, but be nice. Do not mistake your protections as weapons for you to use against your employer or play "I gotcha." If you do, it will work against you. Know your rights, but do not rub your employer's nose in them. Always keep in mind that you need your employer more than your employer needs you. Keep your boss *wanting* to help you in any way he or she can because you are refreshingly honest, likable, realistic, and rational. You will be dealing with individuals, so bring out the best of their capacity to care. If my enlightened approach fails, learn the rules with all their fine details, hold the company responsible, and fight like hell! Here are the major protections and how they work:

Family and Medical Leave Act (FMLA, pronounced fim-la). FMLA is not specifically about disabilities. It is administered by the U.S. Department of Labor and exists to protect us from being fired in the event we need to take time off for medical or other reasons related to the care of ourselves or our families. It has only been around since 1993. It is a blessing. However, only employers with fifty or more employees within a seventy-five mile radius are required to adhere to the act's requirements. Currently, you are covered only if you worked as an employee at the company at least 1,250 hours over the last 12 months. Incidentally, FMLA protects employees when they need to take leave for such things as care of a newborn or care of a spouse, parent, or child. Time off under FMLA, therefore, may protect your spouse should he or she need to take time off to provide your care during an illness. FMLA clearly defines specific requirements for each.

FMLA allows us to take up to twelve weeks of *unpaid* leave a year. It is up to employers to elect how they measure a year, so check their policy. You can use the total allowance of twelve weeks intermittently, meaning that you do not have to use it all at once. Generally speaking, FMLA protects your job as long as you can still perform the essential functions of your job when you return; however, there are some exceptions, such as special rules for "key employees," for example. If you are granted a leave, check with your company about your right to remain on the company's insurance policies (although you pay the costs).

It can get a bit complex because there is an overlap between leaves of absence protected under FMLA and the paid sick and other days (vacation, personal, etc.) you would have earned due to your company's policies. Here's how it works: Although you may *choose* to use paid days you've accrued as part of your leave, your employer may *require* you use those paid days off and count those days towards your twelve weeks. Your employer has to declare if any of your accrued paid time off (vacation, sick, etc.) is being counted towards your FMLA maximum allowance of twelve weeks. Maintain all correspondence and keep accurate records. Companies usually don't cheat, but individuals do.

Be also aware that you can take FMLA leave time in increments shorter than one day. Employers must use the smallest increment their payroll department uses, provided it is no longer than one hour. If you need 2 hours during the day to go to pulmonary rehabilitation for a couple of months, for example, you are allowed as long as it is planned in advance. If the time you request off is "foreseeable," you are required to give 30 days' notice. If you are unsure whether your requested time is "foreseeable" or not, check with your employer or give the Department of Labor a call.

Always remember that many people try to take unfair advantage of FMLA, and human resources personnel are quick to identify them. Be honest, sincere, and forthright. It will pay off.

There are many important "ifs, ands, or buts" regarding FMLA, and laws might change, so if you anticipate taking a FMLA leave, learn all you can about how it works before you apply for it. Visit www.dol.gov/esa/whd/fmla or call 1-866-487-9243 for information.

Americans with Disabilities Act

The Americans with Disability Act (ADA) is nothing less than a powerful piece of civil rights legislation to protect people with disabilities (physical and mental) from discrimination. We have only had it since 1990. It is comprehensive in scope and protects our rights in public and private businesses, local and state governments, public accommodations and services, transportation, communications, and even utilities. Companies with 15 or more employees are required to adhere to this act. The act clearly states that we are disabled if we have a *significant* impairment that limits one or more life activities, such as the ability to care for oneself, learn, work, walk, see, hear, speak, *breathe*, maintain social relationships, etc. Interestingly, this act does not cover people working for the federal government, Native American tribes, or private clubs! Federal employees, federal contractors, and organizations that get federal funds are covered by a similar law, the Rehabilitation Act of 1973. Local and state laws may also protect them.

First, ADA protects us from discrimination when being considered for a job. It protects disabled employees from discrimination in training, promotions, benefits, conditions, privileges, etc. The beauty of this act is that it acknowledges that in order to be treated equally, rights have to be accessible. For example, you can have a sign on the door saying "Everyone Welcome, Walk In," but if the doorknob is too high for some people to reach, the sign has no real value. "Accommodations," therefore, must be made to allow entry to all disabled people so that they can partake of their rights that are available inside that door. Now, a person with a disability might be qualified to do a job, but the accommodations needed for him or her to do the job might be unreasonable to the employer because of undue hardship (usually expense) or other commonsense limitation. An example might be expecting a company to install an elevator just for you. This interplay or overlap between being reasonable and not bankrupting companies (or the local or state government) and being realistically accommodating is called "reasonable accommodation." It is our mantra. If you have COPD, you have the *right* to "reasonable accommodation." Whoopee (if you are reasonable)! There is a fine line between what "reasonable" accommodation is and what is "unreasonable," and how much an employer must adapt to and be responsive to an employee with a disability. It greatly depends on the particulars of the accommodation needed, the resources of the employer, and the physical environment in question.

The Equal Employment Opportunity Commission (EEOC) is the agency mandated under the ADA to protect employees and potential employees from discrimination. If questions arise regarding what accommodations are "reasonable" or "unreasonable," the determination will ultimately be made by the EEOC, which is empowered to bring suit against the employer if necessary. It makes good sense, therefore, to check with EEOC and discuss the particulars of your case. Once again, if you belong to a union, you should go to it for direction.

If you are asking for reasonable accommodation, be specific in your request. It is up to you to identify what accommodations you need, not the employer. It might be wise to discuss your needs with your doctor as your accommodation requests might require medical documentation. Remember to put everything in writing, and don't be insulted when they ask you to "put it in writing."

If you do not work for a company that is required to enforce ADA or FMLA because of its size, you might be at a great disadvantage. However, stay abreast of changing laws regarding labor and entitlements. They may undergo radical changes.

If you are considering changing jobs to one more suitable or accommodating to your COPD, be sure to look at the big picture, including your retirement and/or pension plan, before considering any move to change employers. Remember that you must be well enough not only to get a new job, but to also work for a full year with your new company to be eligible for many protections. When you are interviewed, instead of looking for opportunities for promotion and advancement with the new company, a larger office, more staff, impressive title, or any of the traditional trappings that are important to many people, you should focus on specific working conditions and benefits such as health insurance. Potential employers should not be raising questions about any possible disability. They might ask, however, if there is anything preventing you from doing the job for which you are applying.

If they do ask, don't lie. Generally, the problem is not that there are limitations on what can be discussed; it is just that if something is discussed and you are not given the job, it can be used as ammunition for a claim of discrimination against them (and often is). Interviewers are therefore instructed that certain questions are taboo.

Although you can use FMLA and ADA to enable you to remain employed as long as possible, a day will probably come when you exhaust your entitlements or you simply cannot continue the struggle to work any longer. You may need to retire due to your health. This is probably not the type of retirement you dreamed about. This type of retirement is most often both a relief and a tremendous loss. When this happens, you might need to both maintain your health insurance and find new health insurance (if even available), and plan to live on Social Security Disability and/or other income (or find a more suitable form of employment that is more accepting of your limitations). Incidentally, you can earn a limited fixed amount of money once you are on SSDI and not lose your SSDI, but check with Social Security to determine the current limit and rules. Although FMLA and ADA are important protections, there are some other things you can do to postpone your departure. They require honing your interpersonal skills and working your charm. Voodoo dolls are always an option, but I've had no luck whatsoever with them.

Handle the Little Problems on the Job
Before you get to all the formal ADA and FMLA requests, documentations, etc., you want to buy as much time as you can before resorting to those protections. Buying time often comes down to two things: (1) being able to resolve problems before they become issues of rights or entitlements, and (2) the quality of your interpersonal skills and relationships with those who have power, which means everyone around you—supervisors, peers, and subordinates.

Keeping Your Head Together
Now, I do apologize if I give you the impression that everyone is out to get you. In reality, your supervisors, bosses, peers, and subordinates are just being human. They are not the problem even though they sometimes appear to be. The real problem is your darn COPD; it is interfering with your work, and you are a person with a "disability." It might take time for you to become comfortable with that label. Just remember that even if you work with people who blame you for not being able to keep up, you are not the disease or the cause of the

problem. You have not failed, and you are not a failure. Be proud of what you have accomplished over your many years of work, not just the last few months of it. Your self-respect comes from within, not from the opinions of others who often lack an understanding or appreciation of what it is like to cope with COPD or what it is like to become disabled. Don't expect too much of them; it's hard to know what COPD is like until you've been there. Also, before you leave, don't forget to take enough pens and staples to last you at least fifteen years.

There is life after work. Some "retirees" (forced or otherwise) adapt easily and some find it very hard. People are often surprised how they react, sometimes in a manner very different than they or their family and friends predict. The fact is that you will soon find out that you haven't truly quit working. I'm sorry to have to inform you of this: you have a new job; you are now employed as the full-time case manager for one person, a person with COPD who can probably be pretty ornery at times. So, you thought your last job was hard? Wait! Your first assignment in your new job as a COPD case manager requires that you understand a few things about disability, especially Social Security Disability and Medicare. Get crackin'!

Chapter 7

DISABILITY AND MEDICARE

When one door of happiness closes, another opens; but often we look so long at the closed door that we do not see the one which has been opened for us.
~Helen Keller

Ah, retirement, those precious golden years for which we have worked so hard. Sleeping in as long as we desire, pursuing the finer, slower paced things in life, perhaps some gardening, allowing ourselves to doze off while reading, and traveling—yes, traveling—it's always on the top of the list!

You may have had some of those great retirement years, and they may have been what you anticipated. If you did, count your blessings. Many people are not quite as lucky, but there is a good chance that you can still have many of those finer things you looked forward to in retirement even if you have COPD. Some people become disabled due to COPD after they retire, and some people become disabled, therefore "causing" their retirement. If you are already retired and are receiving Social Security, you will need to understand how your Medicare coverage works. If you are not receiving Social Security, you will need to understand how both Social Security Disability and Medicare work!

Disability means a few different things, depending on who is using it and the context in which it is used. The way we are using it here has only to do with how it applies to collecting your Social Security Disability Insurance (SSDI) due to a serious chronic respiratory illness, COPD.

Types of Disability Insurance
There are three types of disability insurance: (1) private insurance that you purchase or have provided to you as a benefit at place of employment, (2) Social Security Disability and (3) a short-term disability program operated by your specific state.

Private Insurance: If you are lucky enough, smart enough, or successful enough to have private disability insurance and you are not able to continue working, read your specific policy and then contact your insurance company. Policies can vary significantly, from short-term plans that cover you a few months to plans that are in effect for the rest of your life.

State Disability: A few but not all states have programs that provide coverage for injuries that occur *off* the job. Each state that has one operates its program differently. These short-term state-sponsored disability programs usually provide income for only a short period of time. Check to see if your state has short-term disability. Be aware that it is different than Worker's Compensation, which covers you for injuries that occurred at your place of work.

Social Security Disability: Ah, this is the insurance that most readers will find applies to them. It is our safety net. First, it is not a welfare program, so if you think of it as such, please complete the following exercise: Pick this book up to approximately one foot above the top of your head. Next, steady your grip and bring the book down quickly while shouting as loud as you can, "Stupid mutton head!" If it doesn't work the first time, repeat as often as necessary until you've knocked some sense into yourself! Social Security Disability Income (SSDI) is *insurance*. Yes, you paid for it—dearly in many cases! Your benefit amount (money) may vary depending on what you paid in. To be eligible for collecting this insurance, generally (there are important exceptions), you must have worked and earned forty credits (half of these during the last ten years). Although the amounts vary from year to year, most wage earners earn four credits a year. Most people just think of it as having worked full time for ten years, but once again, this is not true for everyone. In any case, always check directly with Social Security to be sure you are eligible. Rules and eligibility can change at the drop of a hat.

If you are fortunate enough to receive SSDI, it is indeed a lifesaver and is not usually taxable unless you have other sources of income that bring you over the maximum allowed. If your other sources of income are too high, you pay taxes only on the excess amount. No doubt, tax rules will change between this moment and when you finish this chapter.

Eligibility for SSDI: Some people think that they are covered by SSDI if they are unable to do their job any longer. *Wrong!* From Social Security's point of view, you are covered only if you cannot do *any* job. Remember that there are many people looking to "get on disability" because they find it too hard or inconvenient to work—you know, setting the alarm clock and everything. Social Security's determination process is set up to weed these people out, and I'm sure there are lots of weeds sprouting. Your need must be thoroughly justified. Justification means your claim has to be verifiable based upon medical records and perhaps examinations by physicians working on behalf of Social Security. They review your medical information, and then follow numbers, formulas, and guidelines to see if you meet the qualifications. This prevents them, as much as possible, from using their own judgment, which, if they did, would inevitably lead to unfairness. Working within the prescribed formula that is provided for them protects them from being beaten on a daily basis by mean-spirited supervisors because they approved too many people. Yet mistakes are made, and there is an appeal process.

Social Security staff follows the agency's "Blue Book" to determine if you are or are not eligible for benefits. The Blue Book is a list of medical conditions and criteria to help determine who gets SSDI and who does not. It therefore pays to be familiar with this book and perhaps check it out before you apply. Some of the main determination requirements are test results, such as PFTs (pulmonary function tests). During these tests, you are tortured with cattle prods and beaten severely while they instruct you to blow as hard as you can into a tube that measures different things about your lungs. I'm kidding, of course; the tests aren't bad, although you might find that you have to let the tester know you need to catch your breath on occasion. Social Security also takes other health issues besides your COPD into consideration. You can review the complete eligibility criteria by looking at Social Security's Blue Book at www.ssa.gov/disability. Once at the site, look for the link for "Blue Book," then "Adult Listings," and then "Respiratory System 3.00." If you think you have a shot of qualifying, you can apply at your local Social Security office or online at www.ssa.gov/applyfordisability. The information they will request is comprehensive and exhausting—often every medication, test, hospitalization, doctor, etc., so be well prepared. Also be aware that you will have to undergo periodic reevaluations to see if you remain disabled. The reevaluations range from filling out a simple form to a full medical evaluation. Because COPD does not get better, the reevaluations are infrequent.

If Turned Down For SSDI

If you are denied SSDI and do not have savings or other ways to survive, such as a working spouse, you may need to apply for local (state) assistance, commonly called public assistance or welfare. If you are notified that you do not meet SSDI eligibility requirements and feel strongly that you do qualify, you can and should appeal. There are various levels of appeal, and you can work your way up the appeals ladder over a period of time—often years. Information on how to appeal is included in your disapproval notification. Many people turn to a disability lawyer upon their first rejection. The attorneys are only allowed to perform their services on a contingency basis and are paid when and if your case is won. Currently (be aware this may change over time), a disability lawyer can only charge 25% or $5,300 (whichever is less) of any back pay he or she helps you get. When you meet with a potential attorney, try to refrain from telling "lawyer jokes"!

Working While on Disability

When you see how much disability money you will receive, please be aware that your convulsive sobbing will eventually subside. You can find out this amount even before you apply by calling your local Social Security office. If you can't make ends meet, one legal option you have, if you have the capacity, interest, and ability, is to work part-time. You are allowed to earn up to a certain amount each month without it affecting your disability income. These numbers change yearly, but it is a reasonable amount. Further, any disability-related work expenses can be deducted from this amount. Social Security actually supports your attempts to work, and it has programs specifically designed to help you. You will find more information at www.ssa.gov/disability. Look for "Ticket to Work" and other work-incentive programs.

Health Insurance Coverage is a Must

We live during times of great change in the philosophy, structure, and delivery of health care in our country. We'll see bills passed, laws created, and regulations enacted. We will then see many years of gradual implementation of those changes, but modifications will be made along the way, and rules changed frequently. No doubt, we'll see backpedaling and politics as usual. Finally, when all this change hits, there is no guarantee that any of the changes will even impact you—although that is unlikely! Nevertheless, it is important that you keep up with those changes. Keeping abreast of changes relevant to your finances and medical care is no small task. Changes in rules that apply such things as Medicare coverage, for example, do not hit the nightly news. You will have to go out of your way to remain current and, hopefully, one step ahead!

Traditionally, eligibility for Medicare health insurance is automatic after you have been disabled (according to Social Security's criteria) for two years plus an additional five month's waiting period (you'll be eligible on the sixth month). This totals twenty-nine months. It is assumed that you have access, during these twenty-nine months, to health insurance under the Consolidated Omnibus Budget Reconciliation Act (COBRA) if other insurance is not available to you. The government has been known to help offset, at times, some of the costs of maintaining insurance coverage under COBRA, but always check the current status. The act was designed with a specific type of individual in mind:

1. Your employer is large enough to be required to provide COBRA benefits. Only companies with twenty or more employees (on 50 percent of its days of operation) during the previous calendar year are required to adhere to this act. The "twenty-employee require-ment," incidentally, can be met by adding up the hours of those who work less than full time.

2. Your employer offers health insurance.

3. You qualify for it.

4. You have savings to pay any costs under the company's group policy or costs not covered by any federal program that subsidizes COBRA benefits.

5. You lost your job for reasons other than "gross misconduct."

Because rules change, be sure to get the most updated informa-tion. COBRA is administered by the Department of Labor, which can be reached at (866) 444-3272 or www.dol.gov. If other insurance coverage options become available, we might see COBRA disappear.

Incidentally, if you are eligible for insurance through COBRA and you are thinking of moving while receiving health insurance under COBRA, be sure that your insurance coverage is transferable, especially if it is out of state, or that other insurance available to you.

If You Can't Afford Health Care or Do Not Have Access to Health Care

If you weren't financially prepared to survive these twenty-nine months, or your life didn't unfold according to the blueprint above and you are without means or medical services, you really should apply for public assistance and Medicaid. They are based on your income and are administered through your state. Every state is different. If your income or assets are too high for regular public assistance but your medical expenses are exceptionally high, you may be eligible for Medicaid's "spend down" or a similar type of program. These programs help you meet your medical costs if they are exceptionally high even if your income is too high to ordinarily be eligible for low-income assistance. In any case, you should check up on your entitlements through www.benefitscheckup.com. Once again, easier or guaranteed access to health insurance might change the rules and how you go about ensuring you have medical insurance coverage, so keep up to date.

Medicare Coverage

First, don't confuse Medicare with Medicaid. People sometimes accidentally use the wrong name, and sometimes they don't know the difference. Medicare is the *insurance* program for "older people" and people with disabilities. If you are deemed disabled, there is no age requirement for Medicare. Medicare is a federal program but is still administered through each state. Medicaid is different. Medicaid is medical assistance for people of very *low income* or resources. Medicaid is different in each state.

You will probably always be allowed to make choices under Medicare. Yes, you have choices to make. Medicare is not handed to you as a complete package; it consists of parts and options. Where there are choices involved, there are advantages and disadvantages to any decision you make. However, choice allows some opportunity to tailor your Medicare entitlements to best suit your individual needs. To make good choices, you must understand how Medicare works and your options. Smart choices can also save you a lot of money. Take the time to fully understand Medicare and your choices. Although the rules are unnecessarily complex, they can be deciphered. As of 2010, coverage is broken down into parts:

Medicare Part A: Covers hospitalization and nursing home care. It has limits, co-payments, and deductibles. This coverage is yours without a fee and is automatic when you get Medicare. Whoopee, pass the party hats!

Medicare Part B: This helps pay part of the cost (usually 80%) of most regular medical care, such as doctor's bills, lab tests, x-rays, and other imaging and medical equipment. Not everything is covered, and there are limits on some things.

Medicare Part C: Private insurance companies offer plans that combine Parts A, B, and sometime D which are paid for by Medicare. Yes, they are private insurance companies but have cut a deal with Medicare to receive Medicare money because they think they can do a better job than Medicare for the same amount of money that Medicare spends directly. They are called "Medicare Advantage Plans." The consumer often (but not always) pays extra for the coverage, and there are many different plans available. The choices available to you depend on where you live. It is also called Medicare Choice. Confused? We'll get back to it in a bit.

Part D: Medicare's drug coverage program, which you have the option to purchase.

Just remember A = hospitals, B = doctors, C = Combo (or Capitalism), and D = Drugs.

If you chose a Medicare Advantage Plan (see Part C above), be aware of the following types:

HMO: A health maintenance organization (HMO) is managed health care with the insurer actually entering a business arrangement with doctors and hospitals rather than just providing payment as do traditional insurance companies. Members use services only within the network, and there is a gatekeeper, a primary care physician who determines your need to see a specialist.

PPO: A preferred provider organization (PPO) is also a choice in a managed care system. It is similar to an HMO except that it covers doctors, hospitals, and services both within and outside of the network (although the coverage is less outside of the system).

POS: Point of service (POS) is similar to PPO, but you have a bit more freedom. You do not need a gatekeeper for care you get outside of the network, but you pay more for that care. You can also stay within the network, get a referral from your gatekeeper, and save money.

Fee for Service: A fee-for-service plan is the most open plan is. For a monthly fee you can go to almost any doctor or hospital, without referrals. The insurance company pays a percentage of the bill and you pay the rest. There are caps on coverage, deductibles, and you may have to pay the bill first and submit it to your insurance company for reimbursement. Sometimes the amount reimbursed is not what the doctor charged. Instead, what will be reimbursed will be a "reasonable" amount (as determined by the insurance company).

PSO: A provider-sponsored organization is new and is not unlike an HMO in that it accepts Medicare payments and accepts full responsibility for the comprehensive care of their patients. Unlike HMOs, which are owned by insurance companies with services provided by those with whom they have contracts, PSOs are owned (at least 51%) by the providers themselves (physicians, hospitals, and other medical professionals).

The policies available to you differ according to where you live—by your zip code, actually. Most areas have a number of companies offering plans and different plans within each company. Generally speaking, you get what you pay for; however, you should only pay for what you use, so you need to review all options carefully.

Medicare Supplement Plans

There are also insurance companies that offer plans that supplement the original Medicare Part A and B plans. If you have a supplemental plan, you do not need any advantage plan (part C). For a monthly fee, these supplement plans enhance what Medicare covers, perhaps more hospital days, picking up deductibles and co-payments, etc. If you use a lot of medical services, joining one makes good economic sense. With these plans, you can go anywhere and to anyone who accepts Medicare. Do not make any choice of a Part C plan without considering a supplemental plan. Although you might see it as pricey at first, if you use a lot of medical services, it may be your best bet.

Do Your Research

Medicare is complex, and frankly I don't know how anyone could review all his or her options and make an informed decision without a computer. Information and help to make informed choices are beautifully spread out for you on Medicare's Internet Web site (www.medicare.gov). Never let any medical coverage lapse without knowing the consequences! If you don't have access to a computer, Medicare will send you the information you need. Currently, you can switch companies towards the end of the year. Once again, start early so you can switch early and get your ID cards in time. Don't assume that the plan you chose this year is the best plan for you next year. Insurance companies often change their plans from year to year, and guaranteed medical coverage might change the way in which Medicare coverage is provided.

Private Health Insurance and Medicare

Many people have private health insurance through their former employer as part of a retirement package or through their spouses. Quite frankly, this becomes confusing if you are eligible for Medicare because you are now entitled to Medicare as well as a private insurance. Speak with your insurance company to figure out how your coverage works with Medicare, and check Medicare's Web site for the latest updates in how such combinations are administered.

State and Local Resources

Remember also that regardless of your coverage (and separate and apart from Medicare), there are state and even county resources that may be available to you if you meet their criteria for being either a "senior citizen" or, in some cases, "disabled." Each state has its own programs (and criteria for each), and the programs come and go. States usually don't spend a lot of money advertising their assistance programs!

Now that you have been introduced to Social Security and Medicare entitlements, kindly remove the hair from your fists before proceeding to the next chapter. Good. You are now in the position of being able to focus more on what you can do to live a good life with COPD. To make the best of what you have, you are going to need good doctors. There is a lot to be considered when choosing doctors, and putting in the time to find the best one for you may be, literally, a lifesaver!

Chapter 8

DOCTORS: EVALUATING, CHOOSING, COMMU-NICATING, AND EXPECTATIONS

Formerly, when religion was strong and science weak, men mistook magic for medicine; now, when science is strong and religion weak, men mistake medicine for magic.
~Thomas Szasz

We must find the best doctors we can. Our lives depend upon it. After we find them, we need to get the best care we can from them. Finding the best doctors and then getting the best care we can from them are two different things. If we just find the best doctors and then leave the rest up to them, it is unlikely we will be getting the best medical care. If that's your approach, you might as well just take the closest doctor and leave it at that. Getting the best medical care requires solid partnering. Just as there are good doctors and bad doctors, there are good patients and bad patients. Find a good doctor and be a good patient.

Understanding Doctors

It is comforting to believe that doctors get into medicine because of a "special calling" and that they are meant to be healers. Although it is true for some, doctors get into medicine for many different reasons—for reasons and motivations as complex as those behind the choices many of us make regarding careers and other major decisions. Consequently, some doctors made the career choice most suitable to their interests, skills, abilities, and dispositions, and some did not. The same holds true for all professions. And yes, there are both great and lousy doctors out there—we've all met some of them, and so have our good doctors. Practicing medicine is not an easy job: sources often cite the high suicide rate of doctors and claim it is over twice the national average. Some doctors graduated at the head of their class and others at the bottom, but the majority graduated somewhere in between the two extremes. Beyond a rich knowledge base and experience, some doctors exemplify great bedside manner and some do not. Because we cannot directly observe their motivation and intellectual prowess, it is not always easy to choose the right doctor. However, if we know what to look for, we can make some sound selections. Although I am trying to encourage you to be intelligent and objective about choosing the right doctors, I fully admit that when you find the right one, you will know it in your gut. There are truly exceptional doctors out there, and it is worth seeking them out. I'm very fortunate; I've found outstanding doctors, but I met some real characters along the way.

Recent scientific studies have discovered that doctors are human, too. We tend not to always attribute all the human characteristics to them, particularly human weaknesses. Frankly, I can "ill afford" a doctor who screws up as often as I do, especially when I'm thinking of one medication but say the name of another (out of a short list)! We want them to be superhuman because we don't want them to be as forgetful as we are, be as distracted as we can be, not get enough sleep some days, have good and bad days like most of us, let their egos get in the way like we sometimes do, and we certainly don't want them to have personal or family problems to distract them! Many of us expect doctors not to have their own problems. On some level, we're better off not knowing about them so we don't have to question their clear-mindedness when it comes to our care. Similarly, most doctors don't want us to see them with all their human foibles either. It is terribly distracting and unproductive. There is wisdom behind this approach and, to some extent, it works. Of course, there are always exceptions.

The Doctor-Patient Relationship

The patient-doctor relationship as we know it has evolved over thousands of years from its origins in healing through magical powers into today's modern medicine. Just like the "old days," faith and belief still have a lot to do with healing and the practice of medicine. Faith in the power of a particular pill might not be required for it to work effectively, but the body as a whole will heal better if we believe it will, and we will even report feeling better if we believe in a treatment. Modern medical practice has not lost sight of this power of belief or faith. It is even factored in when testing new medications.

One thing most of us are in agreement with is that we don't want to be treated as objects. To be fair, however, we also need to be sure we do not treat our doctors as objects either. It is important to re-member that they, too, have needs and weaknesses. They screw up every bit as often as the rest of us and have lousy days and personal problems like the rest of us have. We don't want to have to be aware of those things, and for good reason—we are sick, we need help, and we don't want to have to worry about their needs or if we are catch-ing them on a good or bad day. Many practices are set up to encour-age this distancing; it is a professional distance. What is odd is that we need to be totally open, sometimes naked, and even talk about embarrassing things while the doctor is maintaining professional dis-tance, sometimes clad in a white lab coat. Somehow, it all works.

We expect our doctors to retain a tremendous amount of informa-tion and have quick recall, but the reality is that they see many people each day and simply can't remember everything. They have to juggle a tremendous amount of information while simultaneously attend-ing to patients' emotional needs. You, on the other hand, have to find a doctor with the right balance between his or her clinical skills and a bedside manner that is comfortable for you. If you question people and ask them to rank the importance of bedside manner and clinical skills, they usually pick clinical skills as more important. When they criticize a physician, however, they usually criticize his or her bedside manner. Go figure!

Limitations in Choosing the Right Physician

Some of us might not be in as much control over choosing the doc-tor that is right for us as we would like. Your choice might be limited due to your geographic locale or your insurance. Because you have a serious disease, if there is any way you can maximize your choice of physicians, you should take advantage of it. If you are in a rural area, you might need to drive further than you would like. It is a small sac-rifice. If you have any control over medical insurance, try to *find insur-ance that your chosen doctor accepts, rather than finding a doctor who accepts your insurance!*

Picking the Right Physician for You

Doctors, like Forest Gump's boxed chocolates, come in a variety of shapes, sizes, colors, and fillings (including some nutty and some goo-ey). You may need to poke them a bit to find out more about them. Although first impressions are important when choosing doctors, you will probably not be able to evaluate how good they are until you've seen them a few times. If you have COPD and have a family physician or internist as your primary care physician, you should also see a pulmonologist if at all possible. Some primary care providers are reluctant to refer you to a pulmonologist because they feel capable of treating you. If this is the case, come out and ask directly for a referral, or find one on your own if allowed under your health plan. Be direct with your primary care physician, such as "I would like a referral to a pulmonologist." Don't tiptoe around by asking for a referral in a way your doctor can dismiss, such as, "Do you think I need to see a pulmonologist?" Waiting until you are very sick to start looking for one is not a smart way to deal with your health. When in need, you want to be an established patient and not have to wait months for an opening for a new patient.

The Realities of a Medical Practice and How it Affects Patients

One thing to keep in mind when trying to understand doctors or other medical service providers is that they are often dealing with very needy and sometime desperate people. Here are some things which with they must contend:

1. They have a very stressful job.

2. They are often "on call" for emergencies 24/7.

3. Illness can bring out the worst in people, and doctors have to deal with people at their worst. Some are nasty and blame doctors for just about everything.

4. Some of your doctor's patients are crackpots and call their doctor every time they pass gas. Some even show up, unannounced, with stool samples in a jar.

5. Frequently, doctors trying to be good doctors are also running a complex business at the same time.

6. The average patient seeking ongoing treatment sees his or her doctor probably a bit over three or four times a year, and the doctor treats about twenty patients a day.

7. The average doctor in private practice, therefore, probably sees about 1,400 different patients.

8. Doctors will remember some people better than others, such as those who they have gotten to know over the years, those with unique problems (or personalities), or those who they are actively treating aggressively and with whom they are in frequent contact. Therefore, don't expect too much! The only way to guarantee that you and the finer details of your last examination are remembered is to show up wearing a clown suit complete with curly red hair, red rubber nose, and big floppy shoes. I still get a big smile when I show up, even without my costume.

What to Look for in a New Doctor

1. Wait to get an appointment

It is annoying to have to wait for weeks or even months to get an appointment with a doctor, but it means that he or she is busy. That can be a good sign if there are a fair number of pulmonologists from which to choose in your area. Sometimes doctors limit the intake of new patients, but once in, the doctors are more available to their patients. Having immediate openings is not necessarily a bad sign either. You may have just called at the right time, or it is a new practice.

2. Schedule and availability

Find out the doctor's regular schedule for the office at which you will see him or her. Often, doctors practice between two or more offices and have other commitments. If they are only available to you a day or two a week, that could be a problem unless you can travel to their other offices. Lung infections don't seem to follow schedules very well. Actually, that's not true; they definitely prefer weekends.

3. Parking

The parking should be convenient enough for you to make it from your car to the office during extreme weather or when sick. Don't just think about your current status; plan for the future. Don't take their word for it when you call and ask people on the doctor's staff about parking. They'll usually tell you that it is "right outside" or "very convenient." Something that is "right outside" means something different to someone who gets up early to jog! Take the time needed to actually drive over and view the parking situation for yourself.

4. **Hospital Affiliation**
   If you need to be hospitalized, where would your doctor send you for admitting? You want him affiliated with a hospital in your area with a good reputation. Also, if he is affiliated with the hospital you would use in an emergency, that is to your advantage. In your search for a new doctor, you might want to look through the list of the pulmonologists affiliated with the hospital of your choice. The hospital's Web site often has all the information you want.

5. **School Attended**
   I'm a snob. Some medical schools and residencies are better than others. One of the best Internet sites that provides great information about medical and other schools is *U.S. News and World Report*. It evaluates graduate schools, including medical schools, annually. Go to www.usnews.com and search the site for "Best Graduate Schools."

6. **Patient Feedback**
   There are a few Internet Web sites that allow patients to rate doctors and make comments. You can look up doctors to see what other patients have to say about them. A couple of popular ones are www.ratemds.com and www.healthgrades.com (although such sites are under attack by some members of the medical community). Do an Internet search for "doctor ratings" for more Web sites.

Vital Information Sheet

Before we go further, I would like to introduce you to the "Vital Information Sheet" (also known as "File of Life" or other names). It is a sheet of important information concerning your health and contacts that you can use in emergencies as well as doctor visits. We will refer to it often. Here is one format:

A. Your name, address, and phone number

B. Date of birth

C. Allergies printed in a manner to stand out (e.g., bold or the color red)

D. Emergency contact information

E. Your doctor's names, specialties, addresses, and phone numbers

F. All of your diagnoses

G. All of your medications, including dosage and reason taken

H. Brief statement of prior surgeries

I. Your pharmacy number

J. Insurance information

K. Date that the list was updated (in case you find you have a few different versions around)

Guidelines for Doctor Appointments

There is a bit of a difference in what to expect from your initial doctor's appointment and subsequent appointments. Let me first take a moment to express the importance of *you* also making a good impression! It is imperative that you demonstrate to your doctor that you are realistic, adult, aware, informed, and that you respect and work within the professional boundaries. Dressing well never hurts either.

Your First Appointment

1. **Seen on time**

   You should be seen on time or expect to receive an apology if you were waiting too long. Sure, this might happen occasionally, but as standard practice, it is not acceptable. If they are late because they made themselves available to someone in an emergency, this is reassuring; because there is a greater chance they will inconvenience others when you are in need. If you have to complain, speak up, but don't assume that the problem is the doctor. Often it is the office staff that overbooks. If waiting is a chronic problem, continue to point it out.

2. **Comfortable rapport**

   You should be able to establish a comfortable rapport with the doctor, and you should feel relaxed enough to let your guard down. Remember, they've heard it all and then some. When the visit has concluded, you should walk out of the office feeling relieved, generally good (unless, of course, there was some bad news), and got your questions answered.

There is some possible exception to this rule, however. Some pulmonologists might want you to know from the onset not to expect a cure for your COPD. How they deliver this message is usually uncomfortable, because they often say it in a way that avoids any ambiguity and sets realistic expectations. Don't misinterpret this as a lack of respect of absence of a good rapport. The truth often hurts.

3. **Takes thorough history and does exam**
   This is very important. The doctor should elicit all relevant information concerning your medical history, including illnesses, hospitalizations, current medications, allergies, and how you are currently feeling. Your doctor should also take your height, weight, vital signs, check your throat, perhaps press on your abdomen, and always listen to your lungs and heart. If this is a primary care doctor, he or she should also perform other exams and inquire into other routine things, such as breast exams, prostate exams, stress tests, colonoscopies, etc. You might want to give your doctor a copy of the Vital Medical Information Sheet outlined earlier. A new doctor will ask you about your smoking history. It is valid and important medical information, so don't respond with any of the snide remarks I mentioned earlier.

   If this is a new pulmonary doctor, he or she might want baseline testing done, such as pulmonary function tests, CAT scans, etc., or have earlier ones sent to him or her. One big misconception is that doctors have the time to review reams of unsummarized medical records of prior treatments from other doctors. Ask what records, if any, they want transferred, and don't feel put off it the answer is "none."

4. **Allowed time for intake**
   Doctors usually don't work with just one patient at a time; that's poor time management. While one is undressing, they are with another patient or returning calls. When and if a nurse

comes in to take vital signs, the doctor is often with another patient. Although there might be uncomfortable minutes when you feel ignored, as long as the doctor eventually gets everything from you that he or she needs, you are probably with a good doctor regardless of whether your visit is spaced out a bit. Remember that the nurse is part of the treatment team, is probably human, and almost certainly has a name. Make friends with your doctor's nurse!

5. Elicits questions and listens
   The doctor should be asking a lot of questions. Answer them, and give him or her a chance to ask all questions in an organized manner. If doctors miss something you think is important, you should help them out.

6. Deals with any immediate problem
   Doctors would probably like to get away with just doing an intake or initial examination, because it is enough work; but they should also inquire why you made the appointment and if you have any immediate need that should be addressed.

7. Trust your gut
   Rely upon your instincts to tell you whether you want to put your well-being on the line with this doctor. If you are not sure, try to discern and even articulate what your instincts are picking up. When articulating, try not to do so within earshot of the doctor or staff or give the impression that you are "channeling" a dead relative for advice. Also, muttering your evaluation under your breath while paying on your way out is a bit out of line, too! Do wait until you get home or at least in your car.

Below is a check-off list to evaluate your first visit:

FIRST VISIT EVALUATION

	Great	Good	Fair	Lousy
I was seen on time				
The rapport was comfortable				
The exam was thorough				
A thorough history was taken				
Enough time was allowed				
Important information was elicited				
My questions were answered				
The next appointment was set				
I will feel comfortable to call if needed				
My immediate problem was handled				
I had a good gut reaction				

Ongoing Medical Treatment: What to Expect at Each Visit

The doctor might earn a passing grade during your first evaluation, but you need time to further assess him or her. Be aware that your first appointment is usually taken up by doing an intake. At best, an immediate problem should be addressed, but it won't go far beyond that. Also, if you are presenting multiple problems, your physician might prioritize them and tackle them one at a time. Doctors often do this without explaining or including you in the decision making. You may feel that your doctor is ignoring things when he or she does this, so talk about your "treatment plan" if you want. Sometimes, the treatment plan is as simple as keeping you living as long as possible. You might find that you are seeing the doctor frequently in the beginning, at least until things such as your medications are stabilized.

To help organize expectations, I've broken ongoing treatment appointments down into three parts:

Phase 1: The welcome

1. You are seen near your appointment time or receive an apology or explanation. Although your doctor might occasionally be running late, it shouldn't be the norm.

2. You should be greeted in a respectful, warm, yet professional manner by both the doctor as well as any assistants.

3. You should be escorted to an examination room or office and instructed to remove whatever clothing is necessary. If you are removing clothing, you should be given some type of cover. The assistant should not point at you and laugh as you get undressed.

4. If an examination table is to be used, the disposable cover on it should be new.

Phase 2: Evaluation

1. Your vital signs should be taken and perhaps you should be asked about the reason for your visit if it is not routine. Holding your breath while on the scale is not going to make you weigh less.

2. Your doctor should greet you when he or she enters. Don't expect small talk; it is nice but unnecessary. Frankly, the time can be put to better use unless it is to help you relax. If you are relaxed and comfortable, your doctor might notice this and jump right into the evaluation and treatment. Take it as a compliment.

3. If your doctor starts reading your chart upon entering the examination room, give him or her time to read the notes before launching into your questions. Doctors don't always want you to know that they don't have the same recall as you do regarding your last meeting.

4. Your doctor should ask questions that bring him or her up to date on medications you are currently taking, any illnesses or

treatments, etc. You and/or your primary care doctor have to be your medical case managers. No one else is going to pull it all together for you.

People are often annoyed when their doctor reviews or goes through all their medications each time they have an office visit, even when there are no changes in the medications. Reviewing your medications and other important medical information gives doctors a great overview and refreshes their memory, so let them do their job. You may want to give them a copy of your vital information sheet with your medications on it if it is a long list.

5. Your doctor should inquire about any specific medical complaint you might have or how you are doing in general. This is your time to make the most of the visit. Pull out any notes you brought with you to remind you of thing to discuss with your doctor. You can also use the same notepaper to jot down things your doctor might mention that you fear you'll forget.

6. When beneficial and relevant, you can and should bring the doctor up to date with reminders of your last meeting. If your last visit was routine and did not require follow-through or making any changes, there might be no need to discuss past meetings. If you would like follow-up for something covered at the last meeting and the doctor doesn't bring it up, one standard line that can be used is, "Last time we talked about _____ and I'm wondering if _____."

7. You should have evidence, when relevant, that your doctor is aware of other outstanding illnesses. It doesn't matter if it is from memory or a quick review of your records. If you see your doctors reading your file, allow them time to do so without distracting them with questions. Even after they get to know you well, they may still review your records at the beginning of each visit.

8. When you do ask questions, your doctor should not react in annoyed manner. If you think your questions sound "dumb," remember that doctors are there to treat even us dumb patients. If you don't feel like you can ask questions, you do not have the right doctor.

9. You should not feel rushed, but be aware that physicians need to keep things moving.

Phase 3: Treatment and Follow-up

1. Based upon the evaluation just completed, there should be a discussion, when warranted, of treatment or changes in treatment. If your doctor wants to put you on a new medication, you should receive adequate information about it. It will probably not be comprehensive, just the major points. Your pharmacist will also look for problems—*a good reason to get your meds from one pharmacy!* You can always look up "drug interactions checker" on the Internet, and you will find a number of sites that allow you to list your medications. They will then identify possible problems for you.

2. Check written prescriptions for accuracy before you leave the office. I've known good doctors who constantly either forget to write one prescription when there are multiple prescriptions or do not fill out prescriptions completely. I thought it was just me until I asked around. It isn't just me!

3. If tests are ordered, you should receive a brief explanation of the tests and the reasons for them. Always ask about the follow-up to the tests. Will your doctor call you or should you call in? When?

4. What is the follow-up? Is there anything either of you needs to do before the next appointment? When should the next appointment be scheduled?

5. A pleasant departure is nice and should be expected—be it a hand on the shoulder when going out, a handshake, a smile, or a simple "take care." Always remember to express your appreciation, even if it is a simple "thank you." If it feels appropriate, make the thank you specific, such as "thanks for taking extra time with me today," or "thanks for answering all of my many questions." Now is not the time to say, "Warm up your damn fingers next time!" If the doctor was extremely obnoxious and you know for sure you will never return, feel free to knock on all the exam room doors on your way out and ask the occupants to get completely undressed. Remember to use your most authoritative voice.

6. You should be treated warmly and with respect by the office staff. As a rule, these people work exceedingly hard, and everything they do is in sight of others. They can't stop to clean their ears with Q-tips, stick their tongues out at their boss when they leave

the room, or even take a moment to stare into space without someone watching. It's hard work, so be nice to them.

7. Be aware that much of your contact with your doctor's office might be through a nurse that works with the physician. The nurse is often the one who will report the results of tests, take your call when you are ill, etc. Go out of your way to establish a respectful and appreciative rapport with nurses.

Here is a chart to help you evaluate the appointment with your physician:

Evaluation of Ongoing Doctor Visits				
The Welcome	Great	Good	Fair	Lousy
Seen on time or apologized to				
Greeted warmly by staff				
Clean exam room				
The Evaluation				
My vitals signs were taken				
Greeted respectfully by doctor				
The doctor asked relevant questions				
The reason for appointment was understood				
I was asked about current status or complaints				
The doctor appeared aware of other conditions				
My questions were answered respectfully				
I was not rushed				
Treatment and Follow-up				
Treatment plans or changes were discussed				
Prescriptions were written accurately				
Tests were explained				
Follow-up was planned if needed				
There was a pleasant goodbye from doctor				
Doctor's staff was respectful				

A Special Note

People often report that their doctor told them, "There is nothing more I can do for you." This dismissive statement often brings people to tears. They think of going home to die, but it might simply mean that you are on all the medications and there is nothing more they can do other than help you through flare-ups and to stay as healthy and as functional as possible. If you think about it, that is still doing a lot! If you hear such a statement, you need to ask the doctor to clarify what was said. When you hear such a negative comment, consider the possibility that he or she is expressing his or her own frustration, a reminder for us that doctors, too, are human. You also have the right to speak up if you feel disrespected, but do not stomp out of their office until you put your clothes back on!

No doubt that when you first see a new doctor, especially a pulmonologist, you will be required to get a number of tests. Some of them will be repeated periodically or when there is a special need. You'd benefit by having an overview of the most common tests for people with COPD.

Chapter 9

COMMON TESTS FOR PEOPLE WITH COPD

Treat the patient, not the x-ray.
~ James M. Hunter

There are a few tests you should know about if you have COPD. You will probably have to take some of them. You don't need to know the finer details about these tests, but you should at least be familiar with their names and purposes.

Peak Flow Meter

This little instrument measures how much air you can force out of your lungs in one big burst. It is small plastic tube with a gauge built into it. These instruments are inexpensive and often given out in your doctor's office for you to use at home. Not all doctors use them, and they are more commonly used

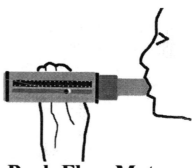

Peak Flow Meter

to assess asthma, which is often a component of COPD.

Pulse-Oximeter

O2 saturation is how much O2 is being carried in the blood. A pulse-oximeter measures both O2 saturation and your pulse. If the O2 in your blood is too low, your organs might not be getting enough O2. The ability of the lungs to absorb O2 is decreased with the progression of COPD, and testing the amount of O2 present in your blood is probably one of the first tests you will have. When tested with the pulse-oximeter, you should be tested both while sitting as well

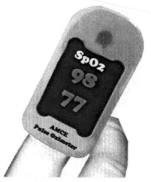

Pulse Oximeter

as when active. We tend to have higher O2 saturation in our blood when we are sitting. Testing is easy. The small pulse-oximeter is placed like a clothespin on your finger and it gives an almost instant reading. The average saturation for a healthy person is between 95% and 100%, and the resting pulse is around 70 beats per minute. Your doctor might use different criteria. Upon activity, a normal person will be able to keep their saturation up, but with COPD we will eventually see our body's O2 saturation start to fall. One test for determining if we need supplemental O2 is to see how we do when moving around. The standard test usually done is called a "six-minute walk test." An oximeter is placed on your finger and you simply walk for up to six minutes to see how far it drops. If it falls below 89% saturation before the six minutes is up, the walk is stopped because that reading indicates that you "should" be on supplemental O2. The "should" is a medical decision and often based, in part, on other things. The "below 89%" is the standard for medical insurance coverage for your O2.

Small Food and Drug Administration-approved portable pulse-oximeters are available for under $70, but can also cost into the thousands. If you are buying one out of packet, simply search under "pulse-oximeters" on the Internet and compare the prices. You will find inexpensive FDA-approved models that are accurate to within 2%. I've tested some cheap ones against pricier ones and found no difference. Some doctors encourage you to use them, and others are almost offended that you dare take on such a thing! Some doctors are afraid that you are going to misuse them or become neurotic. I figure that a pulse-oximeter has never caused anyone to become neurotic; they were neurotic long before they heard of a pulse-oximeter! If you use it for medical reasons, you need a prescription, and it will probably be ordered for you. Your insurance company might cover it, so first check to be sure that it does. If prescribed, you can also deduct it as a medical expense on your taxes. However, be aware that you do not need a prescription to buy one if, for example, you are piloting a small plane and want to check your O2 saturation. Early on in the game, you probably won't need one. They become more important once you are on O2. Don't forget to read all of the literature that comes with your contraption, which should include conditions that may cause a false reading. If you have advanced COPD and are on supplemental O2, talk to your doctor about the possible need for a pulse-oximeter.

Arterial Blood Gas (ABG) Test

ABG stands for "arterial blood gas". The ABG test is a blood test where blood is drawn from an artery, not a vein as we are more accustomed to. Because the blood is taken from an artery, it is fresh from the heart. This allows an analysis of blood before it is circulated and changed by muscles and organs. The tests provide important information about our blood gasses such as O2 and CO2 (among other things). The blood is most often drawn from the wrist area. It can be quite painful or not very painful at all—be ready to curse just in case. I asked one therapist who did painless ones what her secret was and she said that she goes very, very slowly. I was also told by another respiratory therapist friend with COPD (ain't that a kick in the pants?) that you should ask them to use a pediatric gauge needle. The thinner gauges might take longer but they are supposed to hurt less. Feel free to whine like a child if there is no infant gauge available. Drooling, however, is optional.

Six-Minute Walk Test

This test simply requires you to walk for up to six minutes to see how far you can walk before the O2 level in your blood drops below 89% (normal is 95%-%100) as described under "Pulse-Oximeters" above. The test can be used to determine the need for supplemental O2 or gauge your progress or response to treatment.

Pulmonary Function Test (PFT) and Spirometry Tests

The terms "PFTs" (pulmonary function tests) and "spirometry tests" are sometimes confused or used interchangeably, so don't worry about the terminology. Technically, the spirometer is the instrument used to complete a great portion of the comprehensive PFTs, hence the confusion of terms.

PFTs are a series of tests carried out during one session that provides objective information about your lungs. They are usually conducted in a testing lab, sometimes located in a hospital or lab. There are also hand-held portable units that allow a doctor to perform some of the tests during routine office visits. In short, these tests reveal how much air you can move in and out of your lungs, how fast you can move air, lung volume, how well they exchange CO2 for O2, as well as other lung-related measures.

The PFTs consists of tests that require you to blow into a tube hooked up to a machine that collects data. Sometimes the machine (if not the portable ones) is free standing, and sometimes it is part of a small booth you will be asked to sit in. The booth is small and designed with the claustrophobic in mind. You will be asked to inhale and blow repeatedly. Some of the testers aren't too empathetic and you may need to tell them to wait until you catch your breath before continuing to the next test. If you do not blow hard enough or long enough, they beat you with a cat-o'-nine-tails while calling you names that would make the devil blush. Okay, so they don't go that far, but they do push you. A good pulmonologist will want the full PFTs completed when you first start seeing him or her. It will be your baseline. How frequently the doctor wants them repeated depends on the doctor.

In general, you will be told either what "stage" of COPD you are in or some numbers expressed as percentages of lung capacity, such as "you have a 40% lung capacity." There are a whole bunch of tests that comprise a full PFT, but most COPDers tend to only keep tract of a couple of them, at best. The most common test outcomes people tend to monitor are their FEV1 and the DLCO:

FEV1
This stands for Forced Expiratory Volume in One Second. This is how much air you can force out in one second. This is the number that, if you are going to remember only one test number, is usually the number most people think is important. There are standard prediction tables for FEV1 and other tests that compare you with average people to help determine the severity of your lung condition. The results are expressed both in numbers and percentages.

DLCO
This is the lung diffusion capacity test. This measures the lungs' ability to take up O2 into the bloodstream. It is also a gauge of the severity of emphysema in your lungs.

Imaging:
Chest x-rays or CAT scans of your lungs are often done on an annual basis. Comparing images from one year to the next can be important. These tests might also be ordered if you are ill or have shown a significant change in your breathing. Be aware that these scans sometimes

find "things" that are unusual that need to be explored further. This often results (usually unnecessarily) in a "cancer scare." This topic will be addressed in more detail in the chapter on "Common Secondary Medical Problems."

Electrocardiogram (EKG or ECG) or Echocardiogram (Echo)

Cardiograms are painless tests that measure the activities of your heart. They are used to determine the general health of the heart, which includes identifying problems such as an enlarged heart, etc.

Stress Test

A stress test is nothing to get stressed out about! I did everything I could think of to postpone this test because I misunderstood it. It is used to determine how well (or unwell) your heart does when pushed or stressed. There is a long list of cardiac problems the test can determine, and the technician measures various aspects of the condition of your heart and circulatory system. The idea that you are put on a treadmill and chased by a pack of wolves to make you run to the point of having a heart attack is a slight exaggeration. The ASPCA no longer allows them to use wolves. If you can't manage a treadmill, a very common limitation for those of us with COPD, they can inject a substance into you via IV that will get your heart pumping faster while you are lying down and receiving a scan. What could be easier? The substance very gradually increases your heart rate, and it can be stopped at any time and even reversed. Frankly, my heart didn't race any faster than it does when I try to move around on a bad breathing day! They will stop the test long before you are strained to such an extent. Piece of cake! The worst part is waiting to hear the results, but don't let that stop you from trying to get them out of the tester!

There are actually different types of stress tests. One common one is the one described above, sometimes referred to as the dobutamine, persantine or adenosine stress test because of the chemicals injected to get your heart to pump faster. It only takes a short time, usually half an hour. Another type, called the thallium, nuclear stress test or myocardial profusion test, includes injecting a small amount of radioactive substance (thallium) into you. This type of test takes longer because during the test they inject the radioactive substance into you and you have to rest for two or three hours before they resume the imaging. They then turn the lights off and make you run around the room naked while they laugh at the way you glow in the dark. Actually, I found out later that the romp around the room was not a normal test procedure and they came up with it just for me. It was my own fault for falling for it the second time.

Although tests can help figure out what is going on, once your doctor has a clear picture of what is happening, he or she can prescribe the medications that are best suited to your needs. You'll benefit by having an overview of the medications that are out there that are commonly prescribed for people with COPD.

Chapter 10

MEDICATIONS FOR COPD

It should be the function of medicine to help people die young as late in life as possible.
~Ernst Wynder

Along with exercise, proper nutrition, and supplemental O2 (if you need it), being on the correct medications is the most important thing you can do if you have COPD. There is good news and bad news about medications for COPD. First, the bad news: to date, there are no medications available that reverse the destruction of our lungs due to COPD—there is simply nothing available to help us grow new lung tissue. The good news is that it is only a matter of time before there will be medications that reverse the destruction. Headway is already being made! There is always hope that we may be around to benefit from some major breakthrough. Perhaps each new treatment will buy us more time until the next one comes along. There is no doubt that we will, one day, be able to regenerate lung tissue—it's only a matter of time.

One of the most bewildering things is how differently some of us react to the same medication. Although the majority of us react much the same way, some people will report almost miraculous responses to a medication that others swear did not help them at all. Some people have side effects that others don't. Even what turns out to be the best dose and frequency as well as time of day for taking the medications can be quite different between individuals. Figuring out what medications to take and when to take them can sometimes get frustrating and complex; your doctor may give you clear directions or let you play around a bit—such as the time of day you take a daily medication. Further, there might be a periodic need to reevaluate your medications, especially if a new medication is introduced into your regimen or if your disease progresses. Moreover, medications to help your breathing may be affected by other medications you are prescribed to treat illnesses other than COPD. Apparently, the petition we all signed to limit each of us to only one major illness fell upon deaf ears.

Always be aware that on rare occasions, a medication can have a paradoxical effect (which means that the medication has the opposite effect than expected) or you discover you are allergic to it. Always get immediate help if this occurs! Don't go experimenting on your own. *All changes in medications absolutely must be approved by your doctor. Don't increase or decrease the frequency that you take your medicines, the dose, or strength unless instructed to do so by your doctor.*

Medications available or recommended for COPD fall into distinct categories. Generally speaking but not always, individuals are only prescribed one medication from each of the categories. Medications come in different forms: pills, powder inhalers of various shapes, MDIs (metered dose inhalers), and liquid medications packaged in "vials" (or "ampoules" or "respules") to be used in a nebulizer (a small medical device that turns the liquid medication into a mist).

Each of us is unique, and medications might help some people more than others. Only your doctor can determine which medications and what doses are appropriate for you.

The medications you are prescribed to help your breathing work primarily by reducing inflammation and constriction of the airways (although some meds work in other ways). There are different categories of medications and different medications within each category. You are often eventually prescribed a medication from each of the various categories, and it may take a number of trials and errors to get the combination that works best for you. Further, the "reversible" component of our COPD varies from individual to individual, which is to say that medications might help some people more than others. The various medications available are taken at different intervals during the day, ranging from once a day to multiple times a day. Further, some medications are a combination of two different medications, and, to make it more complex, new medications occasionally hit the market! Work with your doctor to find the best medications and combinations and dosing schedule that works best for you.

You will usually find that you have medications that you take every day for maintenance of your COPD and yet another schedule or combination that you need to take when experiencing an "exacerbation."

An exacerbation is a sudden increase in symptoms of COPD and can range from mild to severe. Always alert your doctor to any change in your breathing, amount, quality or color of your mucus, cough, temperature, or any other sign of illness.

New and Improved Medications

New and improved medications are periodically released, and even newer medications are still in clinical trials. Trials, by the way, are not limited to medication trials; new surgical techniques or implements like stents and valves for lungs are also tested and approved in this same way. To track the development of new medications and trials, you will find most of the information you need at www.clinicaltrials.gov.

Warning!

You should familiarize yourself with each medication that you are prescribed by discussing the medication's side effects, contraindications, and warnings with your doctor and your pharmacist when necessary, and most definitely by reading the information sheets available for each medication. You should understand as much as you can about each one and any possible negative interaction it might have with other medications, over-the-counter meds, and herbal supplements. This is especially important in the event you are receiving treatment by someone not familiar with you, such as might occur in a walk-in clinic or nonemergency care center.

Corticosteroids

Okay, I will cover one specific medication, corticosteroids, because COPDers often ask many questions about this particular group of medications. Corticosteroids, often simply referred to as "steroids," are not the same steroids we read about that promote muscle growth in body builders (those are anabolic steroids). Corticosteroids are naturally produced by our adrenal glands and are involved in many of our physiological systems including our metabolism, stress response, and immune and inflammatory responses. Their value for us is their ability to decrease inflammation in our lungs so that we breathe better. The amount prescribed is usually greater than the amount we produce naturally. The medications in this group are synthetic corticosteroids.

Corticosteroids are prescribed in two different ways. The first and most common way is to inhale them directly into the lungs. This is a very low dose, routinely used, and sometimes mixed with other inhaled medications. Corticosteroids are one of the most commonly prescribed medications. They appear to be quite safe, and because of their low dosage, there is even some argument as to whether they even cause or contribute to some of the side effects that occur in larger oral doses (pills) of corticosteroids. Be sure to rinse your mouth and gargle after use, because if you don't, corticosteroids can contribute to oral yeast infections (thrush).

Corticosteroids are also available in much larger doses in pill form (or through IV in hospitals) and are sometimes used for short-term treatment during illness. The amount taken in pill form is usually tapered down slowly unless the treatment is only for a few days. This is done to get the adrenal glands to start producing a sufficient quantity, something they fail to do if synthetic steroids are present in the body for a length of time. It is extremely dangerous to abruptly stop the medication on your own. Be sure to follow your doctor's instructions. Small amounts are sometimes used on an ongoing basis as part of one's daily regimen of medications, although there are many negative side-effects of prolonged use; this is why they are usually used only as a last resort. The time of day they are taken may also be important. In some cases doctors will recommend that they be taken in the morning to stay somewhat in tune with the body's natural cycle of corticosteroid production. At other times, doctors might want to keep the steroid level consistently high throughout the day and want you to take them more than once a day. If you are prescribed steroids, be sure you understand how much to take, how often and what time of the day to take them, and if there is a need to taper. Very short bursts might not require tapering, but it is up to your doctor.

Unfortunately, prolonged oral steroid use has some serious negative side effects, which may include, but are not limited to, swelling and edema (water retention), easy bruising, high blood pressure, osteoporosis, cataracts, acne, thinning of the skin, stomach ulcers, lowering your resistance to infections, raising your blood sugar level, and, of course, suppression of the adrenal glands. They may also interact with other medications. Another side effect of prolonged use is a moon-shaped face and redistribution of body fat, sometimes with a slight bulge at the back of the neck, which, of course, will make you more attractive to camels. Last but certainly not least, even temporary use of prednisone may affect your mood and may, for some people, cause sleep problems.

Medications and Treatments Outside of Standard Medical Care

Although we've talked about medications that fall within standard medical practice, many people look outside of standard medical practice to remedies such as herbs, vitamins, supplements, and potions that may help build up their immunity to infections, protect their lungs, or simply help fight inflammation. We look outside of mainstream medical practice for a variety of different reasons, including desperation. Desperation can change the way we evaluate things. The problem is that most of the alternative products available (yes, I've done a pretty exhaustive search) have not received proper testing. The issue is not only that we might be throwing our money away on ineffective treatments; the bigger problem is that some of the products may even be harmful to us, especially if we are adding them to a cocktail of other chemical substances such as medications!

Just across the border, people from the United States line up as early as 5:00 a.m. to see a doctor who claims to practice live cell therapy—not to be confused with stem cell therapy. The live cells he allegedly injects into you come, supposedly, from the lungs or other body parts of animals. I think he is fond of sheep. He claims that these cells will travel to the lungs and regenerate the lung tissue. His hocus-pocus sometimes includes measuring your chest before and MINUTES after his injections so he can show you how many inches your chest has grown! This kind of makes walking on water rather unimpressive. His practice is largely word of mouth, and his office is flooded with patients, many of whom are there for the second, third, or even fourth time because they believe it works. They are not wackos and, for the most part, are intelligent, serious, and good people. They have not rejected modern medicine, but have added this treatment to their orthodox routine of care. To date, no one (that I know) has grown a tail or started sprouting wool, so the side effects don't appear to be too extreme—hard to believe if you are injecting someone with the live cells from another species! Unfortunately, people believe what they want to believe.

Similarly, a few offices offering stem cell therapy have also opened up in a couple of Latin-American countries. One offers luxurious accommodations at a hotel and private escort service from San Diego across the border. Recently, one of the physicians listed on the Web site of one of these "clinics" removed her credentials after they were discovered to be bogus. Another, I discovered, had his medical license revoked in Wisconsin. There is absolutely no evidence that any clinic outside of the United States has surpassed what has been discovered and accomplished to date by all the legitimate stem cell researchers in the world.

Chapter 11

BREATHING TECHNIQUES AND IMPEDIMENTS

My most underrated bodily function is definitely breathing ...
~ Larry King

What's this, training on how to breathe—something that you've been doing all your life? Yes! There are a few breathing techniques that you must learn if you have COPD. These techniques help us breathe more efficiently and can help us diminish SOB (shortness of breath). These breathing procedures are best taught by respiratory therapists or those conducting respiratory rehabilitation programs because they can provide you with feedback and correction of your technique. If this encourages you to get rehab, good! Because not everyone has access to rehabilitation programs, and because I've known people who have actually attended pulmonary rehab programs and did not get any instructions on breathing techniques (my sister for one), I'll give a brief description of some of the more important ones.

Breathing Techniques
PLB—Pursed Lipped Breathing (or purse lip breathing)
This fist breathing technique is called "pursed lip breathing" because it describes how the lips appear when breathing in this manner. If you watch people after they exercise, you will sometimes see them purse their lips as if they are whistling when they breathe out. Pursed lip breathing is remarkable because it does two things: first, it helps increase the O2 level in your blood; and second, because it can be calming, it can also decreases your need for O2! It is an indispensable technique!

When you purse your lips by bringing them together like you are whistling so that the airflow out of your lungs is limited or constricted, you create a back pressure (resistance) that keeps the airway open and slows the flow of air out of the lungs, therefore helping your lungs do their job more effectively. There should be no force exerted and no stress or strain involved. It should feel comfortable. Indeed, after you practice it for a while, you will find yourself doing it without thinking. People who never heard of this sometimes discover this technique on their own. It is sometimes suggested that you do this for a few minutes a few times a day, but many or most of us do it only when we feel SOB. Yet others of us do it frequently throughout the day without thinking about it.

The technique is:

1. Inhale through your nose (if you can) to the count of one or two, whatever is most comfortable.

2. Bring your lips together as if you are whistling or kissing.

3. Exhale through your pursed lips at a comfortable rate. Do not use extra force.

4. Repeat this and try to exhale twice as long as it took you to inhale. This gently forces more trapped air out of your lungs.

5. After a few minutes, you might find that you can inhale a bit deeper and exhale a bit more. Good. You might want to try to increase the time spent both breathing in and out by a second or two, always trying to breathe out longer than you breathe in. Be gentle.

If you have an oximeter, you will be able to see how well this technique works in bringing up your O2 level. Once familiar with this technique, you might find yourself breathing this way automatically, and in some cases throughout much of the day!

Diaphragmatic Breathing
Babies breathe this way naturally. You can watch their little bellies push out when they breathe, especially when crying. This is also the technique that some people say singers use (probably not true). Some of us even breathe

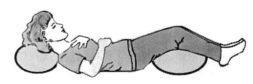

Diaphragm Breathing

this way without instructions or when we are relaxed. Some of us do not. It is an efficient way to breathe because we are less likely to overwork our other breathing muscles.

The diaphragm, which is used in breathing, is a sheet of muscles under the lungs. The diaphragm contracts and then relaxes which creates the pressure needed to suck air into and blow air out of our lungs. Other muscles are also involved in breathing, but allowing the diaphragm to do its job effectively rather than disproportionably relying upon other muscles will help us breathe better. A good way to familiarize yourself with this type of breathing is to do it while you lay on your back with pillows under your head and knees. Try this technique:

1. First, try to relax. Reclining as in the picture below is best.

2. Place one hand over your chest and the other over your belly just above your waist.

3. Breathe in so that your belly expands rather than your chest. You should be able to feel your stomach hand move up and down.

4. Breathing in through the nose and out through the mouth is beneficial, and pursed lip breathing can also be used along with this. It is a great combination!

5. Once you get used to diaphragmatic breathing, you can remind yourself to do it regularly and especially when you seem to be straining your upper torso to breathe.

Huffing or Controlled Coughing

Coughing is a way to bring up mucus from the lungs, but if your coughing is unproductive, there is a technique that might help you bring up stubborn mucus. Controlled coughing lets you get rid of the mucus more gradually than the common cough. It will also help prevent you from stressing yourself out. It is sometimes harder for us with COPD to get the mucus out because we do not have full lung capacity and get SOB too easily. Controlled coughing allows the mucus to take smaller steps rather than trying to expel the mucus in one big stressful cough like we were able to do in our younger, healthier days.

1. While sitting comfortably, place your feet flat on the ground.

2. Lean your head a bit forward.

3. Inhale deeply using your diaphragm and hold it for a couple seconds. Keep your mouth slightly open and cough out twice rapidly but without excess force, you should be doing so by using your diaphragm rather than what feels like your chest muscles. What you are trying to do is give a weak cough, almost as if you are faking one. This technique allows you to replace the strong dramatic cough with shallower, more numerous coughs to slowly get the mucus from the lungs. If it is yellow or green, has changed in consistency, there is more mucus than usual, or it has blood in it, you should alert your doctor.

4. After resting a bit, repeat step 3 until the mucus is discharged. Be patient. The whole point is to do it slowly without stressing or straining yourself. It is like taking small steps instead of large strides.

Be aware that mucus often slowly works its way up on its own without coughing, so sometimes just giving it a rest of a few minutes between controlled coughing eventually leads to a productive cough. Be sure to keep your body well hydrated, which will help thin your mucus. If thick mucus is a chronic problem for you, talk to your doctor about taking something to thin the mucus.

General Tips to Help You Breathe
Pacing your physical activities properly has a lot to do to with preventing SOB. Many of us rush to get something done only to experience the distress of being SOB once we reach our destination. Slow down! It is better to walk more slowly and even stop to catch your breath before you are short of breath.

Sometimes sitting with your feet flat on the floor and relaxing your shoulders and back muscles by letting your head drop downward while relaxing your hands, palms upwards, will help you relax and catch your breath. Don't forget your PLB (pursed lip breathing) and diaphragm breathing while sitting in this position. You can also sit with your head forward on a pillow placed on a table. Don't forget to relax your arms and shoulders. If standing, you can rest, slumped over a bit, with your arms resting (not ridged) on a counter. Another alternative when standing is that you can place your back against a wall for stabilization while standing with your feet slightly apart. You can then relax the shoulders and let your head drop forward a bit— again while doing PLB and breathing through your diaphragm. The concept behind all of these techniques is to help you relax, especially your shoulders, and to not demand more energy. If you can, have a professional respiratory therapist teach you these techniques.

Air Quality and Breathing

Air quality can affect your breathing, be it indoor or outdoor air pollution, smog, fog, humidity, temperature, etc. Further, seasonal pollens and other allergens might affect you even if they've never been a problem before. For most of us, our lungs simply become very sensitive. Occasionally, our weather service will announce a smog alert, hazardous air, or pollution alert. Pay attention to those days, and try to stay indoors in an air-conditioned environment.

One thing most of us notice is that our breathing is affected by such things as perfumes, odorizers, deodorizers, and many of the smells used in household products. It seems that anything that has a smell, pleasant or unpleasant, bothers our breathing. Find ways to avoid anything that irritates your lungs.

You might also find that in addition to outdoor pollution and indoor smells, pets and animals bother your breathing. This is very individualistic and is something you should discuss with your doctor if you are a pet owner.

Air Purifiers

One way to improve indoor air is to use an air purifier. There are reports (American Lung Association, Environmental Protection Agency) that ionizing or ozone-producing air cleaners (or electrostatic precipitators) can aggravate asthma and COPD symptoms, or worse, even permanently damage lungs. It might be wise to stay away from any air purifying device that refers to ozone, ions, or ionizing air without first checking with your doctor. Many of us find that a good mechanical filter is the preferred way to go, and the best filters are reported to be HEPA (high efficiency particulate air filters) because they trap extremely fine particles. Before buying a filter, check to see what size room they will clean. Some of the smaller ones only clean very small rooms. Some filters also have charcoal filters in addition to mechanical filters. The charcoal will absorb even finer impurities in the air. Charcoal filters tend to be a bit costly. In any case, check to see how long the filters will last, how much it will cost to replace them, and if replacement filters are readily available.

COPD is all about breathing, and the techniques will no doubt help you. When techniques are no longer sufficient to provide you with the O2 you need, your doctor will probably prescribe supplemental O2. You may already be on supplemental O2 or it may be far down the road; but if you need to use it, you will need to understand it.

Chapter 12

USING SUPPLEMENTAL OXYGEN

"Air is like sex; it's not important unless you aren't getting any"
~Anonymous

Supplemental O2 (oxygen) has been consistently proven to prolong life and improve the quality of life for people with COPD. It can significantly increase your ability to walk, exercise, and even to have sex! O2 is so good that…well, they bottle it!

We need O2 to live. Because our lungs are damaged, we cannot fill our lungs with the amount of air we need or absorb the O2 out of the air as effectively as we did before we had COPD. If we can't pull O2 out of the air like we used to when we were healthier, then we need to increase the amount of O2 in the air we breathe. Most of us with COPD will end up on supplemental O2. Needing supplemental O2 simply means needing more O2 than is available naturally in the air. You will only be prescribed O2 when tests show that you need it to maintain a sufficient amount of O2 in your blood. To get more O2 into our lungs, we use tanks of liquid or gas O2 or machines that produce O2. We inhale that O2 through a hose and nosepiece called a cannula. This hose that goes from the air supply to the nose is also called, sarcastically, a nose-hose. No one *wants* to be on supplemental O2, but when you do begin to use it, you will "come of age" and become a member of an exclusive group. Although people often kick and scream about using it, sometimes swearing they will never use it, once you become acclimated to using supplemental O2, you will wonder what all your earlier fuss was about; yes, it is inconvenient, but it is really not all that bad. There is a lot of misinformation about O2 for people with COPD, so we'll start with a couple of myths.

1. **Myth: You will be dangerous and blow up friends and family.**
   Fact: O2 is safe as long as you follow some simple rules. If O2 were flammable, which it is not, our atmosphere would be on fire like the sun. I think that would be a tad uncomfortable. In

fact, O2 is not flammable. The confusion lies in the fact that fire needs O2 in order to burn; O2 is an "accelerant." Fire uses something else as fuel, but needs O2 to burn the fuel, and the more O2 it gets, the quicker it is to ignite, and the hotter and faster it is able to burn. Remember, firefighters wear O2 gear into fires (however, they have other protective gear and special training). On the other extreme, every year people using O2 set themselves on fire because they are careless. Most of them are smokers using O2.

2. **Myth: People will stare at you and make you feel uncomfortable.**
    Fact: Most people couldn't care less and won't even hold a door open for you! I could give you many anecdotes of people resisting using their O2 in public, but the stories are all the same: They resist, give in just a little (maybe just to the doctor's office at first), test the waters where there are few people around, slowly increase using supplemental O2 in public, and, when they see that no one gives a darn, they eventually find that they are no longer self-conscious. I can all but guarantee that within a short time, you will be comfortable, forget you are using it, and will be able to look back at how "silly" your fearfulness was.

    Children can be an exception. They are more curious about the world around them and notice more than most adults. They are certainly less censored in their reactions. They may stare, giggle (not as in laughing at you), squint, ask, or otherwise express curiosity. What a wonderful opportunity to encourage and reward their curiosity by talking to them, even if you have to initiate the conversation. Your 30 seconds of explaining your O2 might be the most meaningful (and educational) part of their day, and they may remember it for the rest of their lives. One friend on O2, while shopping using an electric cart, got separated from her granddaughter. When someone tried to help her granddaughter, she described her missing grandmother as "riding in a cart with something hanging out of her nose." Kids can be amusing, but their parents are not always that comfortable about their children's curiosity and may discourage their interest and attention—all because they want to be polite. Let them know you enjoy explaining such things to children and they are lucky to have curious kids—regardless of how expensive they are to feed.

3. **Myth: You will become dependent on it.**
   Fact: We were all born dependent on O2! Using supplemental O2 keeps the level of O2 in your body up to the amount your body was designed to require. Not having enough O2 is extremely harmful. You body does not become dependent on it like a drug or make it harder to go without it.

4. **Myth: Your lungs will become lazy.**
   Fact: If you are not getting enough O2, you probably are not as active as you could be; therefore, your whole body isn't getting proper exercise! Actually, your lungs and heart are experiencing quite the opposite of laziness. If they are not getting enough O2, they are becoming stressed because they are overworking! With supplemental O2 you can give them a break and exercise them properly rather than stress them. There is a myth about people getting "lazy lungs" once they start using supplemental O2, and it probably came, in part, from a real phenomenon that exists with a small number of people who have a problem getting rid of CO2 (carbon dioxide). This complication will be explained shortly.

Oxygen in Nature
In nature, O2 is a gas, but not a liquid gas like gasoline (although O2 can be made into a liquid by some fancy distillation and condensation). First of all, the air we breathe is a mixture of things; it isn't all O2. As a matter of fact, only about 21% of the air (at sea level) is O2. Most of the air we breathe is made up of 78% nitrogen. The balance is made up of carbon dioxide (CO2), argon, trace elements, and a variable amount of water vapor.

Oxygen as Medication
Think of O2 as a medication and a medication delivery system. It needs a prescription, dose, strength, etc. There aren't many things you can do for COPD, but using supplemental O2 when needed is one of the most important. It is not going to restore your youth or mask your disease, but that should be no excuse not to use it. The reason you use it

is to increase the O2 available to your body, which includes your organs. The results of organs trying to function with inadequate O2 are very injurious and can lead to organ failure. Often, an organ tries to compensate for the lack of O2. The heart, for example, might become enlarged, or the quality of your blood might change to make up for the lack of O2. There are serious and potentially deadly consequences of not using O2 when it is prescribed.

When You Need Oxygen

The most common way to establish the need for supplemental O2 (there are other ways) is to conduct a test called the "six-minute walk test." You will walk (without O2 at first) for up to six minutes, or until your O2 saturation is at 88% or below, whichever comes first. If your O2 saturation dips below 88%, you might need supplemental O2. If you are able to walk for six minutes without it dipping below the 89% saturation point, you do not need O2, according to this standard (unless other medical conditions exist, such as congestive heart failure, etc.). Some doctors are not concerned if it drops below 89% for a bit as long as it bounces right back up; that short drop, they say, will not harm you. Others like to keep the numbers higher at all times. How much O2 you need and when you need it is up to your doctor to decide; you might need one amount of O2 for sitting, another level for activity, and another level for sleeping. The amount prescribed is measure in LPM (liters per minute). Commonly but certainly not always, people first start using supplemental O2 at night while sleeping because it is normal for the blood O2 level to decrease while sleeping because our breathing is shallower. Be aware that although your SOB might be so severe that you are convinced you need supplemental O2, tests may indicate otherwise.

Danger of Too Much Oxygen

People are warned, for good reason, not to adjust their O2 on their own and to stick with their doctor's orders or instructions. The reason for this is that the lungs' work is twofold: first, absorbing O2 into the body, and, second and equally important, expelling CO_2 from the body. There is a risk for some people, but not all people, that increasing the amount of O2 too high might reduce their impulse to breathe deeply or often enough. This could lead to a buildup of CO_2 in individuals who lack the triggers to breathe more rapidly and/or more deeply when there is an excess of CO_2 in the blood. If CO_2 is allowed to build up, the elevated level of CO_2 remains in the bloodstream and can result in rapid heart rate, seizure, respiratory arrest, coma, and death. This is not a problem for most of us, although we may develop this problem when seriously ill. However, there are exceptions, and everyone who uses O2 needs to follow his or her doctor's recommendations. People who have a problem ridding their body of CO_2 are referred to as "CO2 retainers" or simply "retainers." The most accurate way to determine if you are a retainer is to have the level of the CO2 in your blood determined. Incidentally, keep your eye out for nimble-fingered children who like nothing more than to play with knobs on a supplemental O2 apparatus. They might inadvertently be adjusting your O2 for their amusement. Of course, if you turn bright colors as a result, it simply adds to their entertainment.

Get the Training You Need

I'm making no attempt to tell you everything you need to know about using supplemental O2. Unfortunately, doctors seldom provide training, and they leave it up to the O2 supplier. Some suppliers do a great job training consumers and some don't. Speak up to be sure someone trains you properly. You should minimally be aware of how to:

1. properly use and maintain your equipment;

2. properly use tubing and cannulas, including how often to replace them and how to get replacements;

3. use your O2 backup system in the event your primary system fails;

4. how to prevent problems by ensuring you have all the equipment you need, such extra tools to turn valves on portable tanks in case one breaks, a gasket for your portable system (if used), and batteries, if your portable system uses batteries;

5. understand requirements for safe storage of all O2 equipment.

6. complete O2 safety training.

Types of Oxygen Delivery Devices

This is a tricky subject for a few different reasons. First, new and better systems of O2 delivery are being invented all the time. Second, insurance companies do not embrace the more expensive (most often newer) devices, and third, reimbursement from Medicare, Medicaid, and medical insurance companies to vendors limits what options they make available to us. Because of the politics and money involved in supplying O2 to us, things are constantly changing. Consequently, what is "available" theoretically might not be what is actually "available" to you. If you have the financial means, you may be able to afford the most advanced portable concentrators and flaunt them within our COPD crowd—it's our equivalent to a Rolex watch.

Oxygen Concentrators

Concentrators are electrical appliances that provide a continuous flow of O2. Portable O2 concentrators are discussed below. They take room air and increase the O2 level by removing nitrogen. The O2-enriched air is then inhaled through a cannula, which is a hose with prongs that fit into the nostrils. The amount of O2 provided is adjustable. They can run 24/7 with periodic servicing and require frequent cleaning of the air filters. They are primarily used around the house or where there is an electrical outlet, such as in hotel rooms and some recreational vehicles. Rather than jumping up and down to change the flow (amount of O2), some people have inserted a "flow regulator" between their cannula and long hose. They can't be used with all concentrators and might cause damage to some. One place I've seen them is at www.softhose.com, and they are listed under "flow control valves."

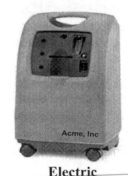

Electric Oxygen Concentrator

Becoming more popular, especially with O2 supply companies because of the cost savings, are O2 concentrators that function as not only as regular concentrators as described above but also have the extra advantage of being able to refill small, portable O2 tanks at home. These concentrators are called, aptly, "home-fill systems." Although you might like the convenience of being able to fill small O2 canisters in your own home, you might only get a limited number of refillable canisters, so the amount of time you can be away from home is often a problem.

Portable Oxygen Concentrators

There are also portable concentrators available that can run on house current, plugged into your car's power outlet, or used with portable rechargeable batteries. Most are allowed on planes. If you are thinking of getting one and like the feature of being able to plug it into your 12-volt car power outlet, check the owner's manual for both your car and the concentrator (always available online) to be sure your car produces the adequate watts.

Pinching the Pennies

Some localities offer discounts from the electric companies if you are on O2 concentrators or other life support equipment, so check with them to see if you can get a discount. Even if they do not offer a discount, registering with them might help prevent them from shutting off your service as well as give you preference in the event they are responding to a blackout. Incidentally, it is still illegal for someone to murder you because of nonpayment of a bill. In the event your electricity is turned off or your O2 equipment removed because of nonpayment, and your health is compromised, call 911.

You may be able to take the cost of the electricity used to operate your electric concentrator as a medical deduction on your taxes. Check with your tax preparer to see if you can take this deduction and if it would be beneficial for you to do so.

Cannulas

Ask your doctor how often you should change your cannula. Most O2 suppliers will provide you with enough to change it every two weeks. I buy extras out of pocket. Most people prefer the soft cannulas. Ask your supplier about them.

They often have a chemical smell to them when first opened, so many of us let them air out a day or so before we use them. Most people wear them with the prongs arched up, but this bothers some people if it rubs the inside the nostrils. If this happens, some people cut the prongs down to make them shorter. Others turn them upside down so that they are arched down instead of up, but still within the nostrils. As long as

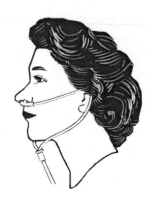

Cannula

you are getting the O2 in (be sure you are), it isn't a problem. If you have an electric concentrator, most will instruct you to limit your hose length to 50 feet or less. My vendor supplies me with a new one every three months, but I have to ask.

Oxygen Gas Cylinders

Bottled under pressure, theses cylinders have concentrated O2 gas and are probably the type with which you are most familiar.

They are commonly used and come in a variety of sizes, from ones that fit in a knapsack to ones so large that they resemble (for lack of a neutral description) huge bombs. There is a valve to open and close them. There is a "regulator" that fits over them so you can regulate the amount of O2 released. Do not allow air to be re-leased from a tank too quickly, such as when purposefully emptying a tank.

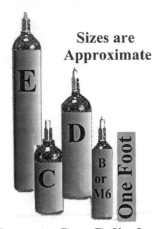

Oxygen Gas Cylinders

Conservers: Pulse Dose (On-Demand) Regulators

Small devices called "conservers" are available that fit onto the re-lease valve of gas O2 tanks (above) that help lengthen the amount of time a tank will last. The ones that work on gas pressure and do not use batteries are called "pneumatic" types. Those that work using batteries are called "electronic." Here's how they work: Ordinarily and without using a conserver, the O2 is released in a constant flow, although you can adjust the flow amount (by liters per minute or LPM) with a regulator. This means O2 continues to leave the tank even when you are exhal-ing. This O2, unless you are inhaling, is wasted and the tank runs out of O2 rather quickly. A conserver works by only releasing the O2 when it senses that you are

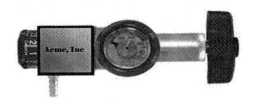

Oxygen Conserver

inhaling and shuts off the flow of O2 when you are not inhaling. The O2 comes out in "spurts" or "pulses" and is often audible. It works by detecting the change of air pressure when you breathe through your cannula. Some models give you a "spurt" every time they sense that you inhale, and others are set to give you a spurt on every second or third inhalation, depending on the setting. Some people can't use the on-demand dose (spurts) and find it best to use the continuous flow because it allows them to adjust their breathing, both the depth and frequency, as needed. Others get along by just adjusting the flow more frequently.

If your conserver on your portable O2 system is battery operated, you should always have spare batteries with you at all times. Although some batteries might last a bit longer when refrigerated, they may also need to be warmed up before use, so *do not refrigerate your backup batteries*, just be sure they are relatively fresh. Also, if you are carrying more than one portable tank, be sure that the backup tanks actually have O2 in them. My company enjoys sending empty tanks regularly. Also have your O2 supplier show you where the "O" ring on your conserver is and ask for extra ones in case it falls off. If your "O" ring goes missing, your conserver will not work.

Liquid Oxygen (LOX)

Liquid O2 (LOX) is made by removing the carbon dioxide and water vapor from air, condensing it, and slapping it around to make it a cold liquid. Because it is concentrated, you get a lot more O2 compared to O2 gas (by both the volume and weight). The advantage of being able to carry more O2 with the economy of less space and weight makes it very popular with experienced COPDers, because a full portable tank lasts you a rather long time compared with the gas cylinders. One brand says their 3.6-pound portable tank lasts up to ten hours, depending on the dosage. Its drawback is its expense and possibly its availability, because, once

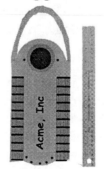

Size Approximate

Portable Liquid Oxygen Unit (LOX)

again, of the politics of insurance reimbursements. When something is more expensive, availability and coverage become issues. The small portable units can be refilled from a larger tank stored in your home.

Just hitting the market are home-fill units for liquid O2. These are units for home use that work like regular concentrators, yet make liquid O2 for your portable units. Similar units for making and filling gas canisters have been around for a few years, but these liquid producing units look very promising!

Ordering Equipment and Choosing Vendors

I bet you thought making arrangements for your O2 would be taken care of by your doctor, didn't you? In many cases it will be taken care of by your doctor or the doctor's staff, but you need to ask a few questions to see if they are on the ball. Often, your doctor will order "concentrator for home use and portable O2." That's it. The vendor will try to get away with the cheapest combination available and may not even ask questions about your lifestyle or activity level before showing up with what *he or she* wants you to use (always the cheapest). Take control and be ready to do some self case management. Be the liaison between your doctor's office and vendor.

What I did find over the years of discussions with other COPDers was that their satisfaction (or dissatisfaction) with the various companies that provide O2 seems to differ widely. Some people swear by small local companies, and some like the nationwide companies. Regarding the large national companies, I have come to the conclusion that how the branch office is run is more important than the name of the company. Because of this, it might be best to take your doctor's advice in picking a vendor. They will know the local companies and which ones are easy or difficult with which to work.

Storage of Oxygen Gas

Discuss proper storage of O2 canisters and all safety precautions with your O2 supply company. Make the vendor do its work. Play dumb and ask a lot of questions. If you start showing off how much you already know, the company might hold back. I'm not going to pretend that I am covering all the safety information and rules; as a matter of fact, I'm warning you that I am not! Besides, I've gotten some conflicting information over the years. What I have learned is that O2 canisters or tanks

Pickup Before: 11/2/2012

GOODWIN

3270

need to be stored in well-ventilated areas, because escaping O2 gas could saturate the area and make it dangerous. Tanks should be stored upright or on their sides in a manner that prevents them from sliding around or knocking in*~ Milk crates are commonly used.

platform. Tanks should never be
;! Remembering that heat makes
direct sunlight or heat, such as
ecause the pressure in the cylin-
ld that there is supposed to be
e should the pressure exceed a
fy this. Also, there is a problem
ap-seal valve could break and
herefore, tanks should be se-
left to roll around. Remember
pposite the release valve, so
be seated accordingly.

nner as pressurized O2 gas
t is liquid, the liquid is cor-
all the "do's and don'ts" and
"freezes." If you use liquid,
liquid spills on you, your

If .... use any oil or grease on your O2 equip-
m..... yourself, including your nose.

Oxygen, Nostrils, and Humidifiers

Dry nostrils and sinus problems plague O2 users. To help keep the membranes from drying out, humidifiers are available that hook up to your O2 concentrator. They require diligent cleaning and disinfecting as per the manufacturer's instructions. Instructors often fail to provide adequate training on proper cleaning and disinfecting of the humidifier that attaches to concentrators. They also often neglect to inform the consumer that distilled water is recommended. House or room humidifiers might also help; just be sure to keep them disinfected.

There are OTC (over-the-counter) water-based nasal moisturizers and saline solutions available at your pharmacy to help dried nostrils. Don't use oil or petroleum-based products around O2, including in your nostrils. Keeping your nose, sinuses, and throat area healthy is important. If they are not kept healthy, they are more prone to infection, and those infections can travel to the lungs. Also, oil- and petroleum-based products are not good to use in your nose because small oil particles might travel to the lungs and cause serious problems. You have enough lung problems already.

Other Useful Things

There are a few useful things available that might help make O2 use easier for you.

Water Traps

Water can condense in your hose due to temperature changes, especially when the hose is on the floor. Your O2 company can give you little "water traps" to collect the moisture. Some companies won't tell you about them unless you ask.

Swivels

Generally speaking, your hose should not be longer than 50 feet (or less if the manufacturer says so) or the pressure to push the O2 through the tubing will be compromised. You can attach swivels, small plastic devices, between your cannula and tubing or between sections of tubing to help prevent some of the tangling. You'll probably have to ask your provider for them. Once again, they may not be offered without asking.

Carry Bags

There are a plethora of bags available to carry your small O2 tanks, be they gas or O2. Some hold multiple tanks, some bags fit over the arms, some are worn as backpacks, and some even as fanny packs. If you search for "oxygen cylinder bags" on the Internet, you'll find numerous choices.

Tubing and Hoses Everywhere!

Tubing and cannulas can be a problem. The darn things get stuck in refrigerator doors, under chairs, or otherwise where they shouldn't be just so they can cause you to trip. They are undoubtedly possessed by Satan and have a mind of their own. Whenever someone trips on a hose, a devil gets his wings! The act of accidentally tripping on the darn things creates a constant hazard. Know where your hose and cannula are at all times, and if you need to keep them off the ground, there are small plastic or metal hooks that can be affixed to a wall or appliance, such as a refrigerator, to hold the hose off the ground. To deal with the mess of tubing, there is at least one manufacturer of a retractable reel for O2 tubing, www.oxy-reel.com.

Transtrachael Systems

Transtracheal oxygen systems (TTOs), consist of putting a catheter through a small hole in the trachea (windpipe) through which the O2 travels to the lungs. This requires making a small hole in your throat area. One advantage of the system is that less O2 is required and the supplemental O2 bypasses the nose, sinuses, etc., which can be a major sources of irritation and problems for some people, especially those of us on higher O2 settings. There are also some cosmetic advantages because the catheter is concealed by your clothing and you don't have to wear an O2 cannula in your nose (but you will still have to carry a small tank of O2). The procedure is not that involved, and patients are usually released the same day it is put in. Weekly follow-up is required until your body gets used to it. It requires daily cleaning and maintenance at home. With the scoop, there is a risk of infection and a buildup of mucus balls. I've known a few people who had it done, and almost all were very pleased.

Safety Around Flames or Sparks

Again, O2 is not a fuel, but it feeds a fire. Be aware that if there is a fire directly in front of you with the O2 feeding it, there is the awful possibility that the flames and smoke could be inhaled and travel down your windpipe into your lungs. You couldn't ask for anything worse to happen, and we've all read of these catastrophic events, usually to someone smoking while wearing O2. It is a nightmare, but you can put your nightmares to rest by following some simple rules and changing your habits.

You must be very careful around flames, sparks, etc., when using O2. It is consistently recommended to have your O2 source ten feet from flames or sparks. Therefore, don't be sticking your head or nose into a water heater to see if the pilot is on! Where there is a chance of a spark, there is a chance of fire, and even a single spark could ignite a fire if the immediate atmosphere is enriched with O2. The area immediately around your cannula is one of those enriched areas because not all the O2 coming out of the cannula is inhaled. Further, your cannula itself could melt and burn (and release vinyl chloride fumes or other substances) while being fed a continuous supply of O2. Worse, this could all be happening right in your face! O2 users are also advised to stay away from appliances that might spark or appliances that get close to our face, such as hair dryers and electric shavers.

Kitchens are one of the most unsafe areas because of the sparks, flames, and volatile oils, such as cooking grease. That little potholder fire, singed hair, or minor grease fire that most of us has had in the past could quickly become life threatening if you are using O2. It is advisable to prepare all your food, and then, if possible and with your doctor's approval, remove your O2 temporarily while attending to a pot on the stove. This can sometimes be done while sitting. Both electric and gas stoves are dangerous. Some people disregard the warnings and continue to cook on a stove but do so very carefully. They wear their cannula from the back like a ponytail, over the ears and then into the nose. In doing so, they are taking a big risk. If you are able to negotiate a bit of cooking without your O2, or use a microwave, you will find many cooking and kitchen tips later.

Traveling with Oxygen
Yes, you can travel with portable O2! O2 suppliers are prepared (or should be) to load you up with the extras you need to travel. I've even known people who have traveled to Europe on O2! Just remember that the higher elevation you are, the less O2 there is in the air, and you might need to compensate for that difference by increasing your O2 according to your doctor's instructions. If you are using an electric or portable O2 concentrator, your machine itself might have limits regarding working at higher altitudes, so check your owner's manual.

You will find many travel tips in a following chapter on "Getting Out, Mobility, and Travel"; however, here is some additional information for the supplemental O2 user.

Driving
You can drive using O2. Be sure to secure your O2 tanks properly, and don't forget spares. Also be aware that some of the smaller

electric portable O2 concentrators can be used with a battery or plugged into your car's power outlet. Yes, you'll see that your car is probably a 12 volt and assume they work in yours, but also check your car's amps or watts produced against how much your concentrator requires. You will find this information hidden in the owner's manuals. Further, if your engine is large enough and the electrical system appropriate, you can have your mechanic install an AC converter in your car.

Be aware that when traveling, you can often plan in advance to have your O2 tanks refilled along the way; however, it requires careful planning and a company that has offices along your route. Although larger companies are better prepared to handle such requests, check to see it this is available if you use a smaller company. Many smaller companies work with each other.

RV Travel
What a way to travel, especially if you can afford a motorized Class A vehicle! A Class A motorized vehicle has the living area within the same area as the driver and passenger seats. Most come with electric generators. This is great for your O2 concentrator, because you can plug it in when on the road and also sit up front if you choose. Unfortunately, laws regarding recreational vehicles that fit over the truck cab (pop-ups, fifth wheels, campers, etc.) or that require towing do not allow passengers in the living area when they are moving.

Rail Travel
Trains are actually a good way to travel for people who use O2. Travelers have praised Amtrak for its service and accessibility (but complained about delays). There is a limit on how much O2 you can transport. Contact Amtrak at www.amtrak.com (800-872-7245).

Commercial Bus Travel
You can travel with O2 only if it is for use during travel (not transported as luggage) and you make reservations informing them of your O2 use in advance. There are different companies and they have different rules, so call the bus company you plan to use. Ask for the person who answers questions about traveling with disabilities, rather than the first person who answers the phone.

Air Travel with Oxygen

Always discuss your travel plans with your doctor before making any travel arrangement. If you do not ordinarily use supplemental O2, you might need O2 when flying. If you ordinarily use O2, you might need more O2 than usual while flying because the pressurized atmosphere is not what we are used to at ground level. In any case, you will need your doctor's cooperation to make necessary arrangements.

Although we cannot be denied access to regularly scheduled air travel, including boarding assistance mandated by the ADA, the issue of traveling with O2 is a bit more complicated. It can be and is done, sometimes without a snag—and sometimes it turns into a disaster. There are a number of different things of which you must be aware if you plan on traveling by air with O2:

- You cannot bring O2 on board the plane or pack it in your luggage.

- Although most airlines used to make arrangements for O2 on board (you had to use theirs, not yours), most airlines now require passengers to use portable O2 concentrators. They usually don't let you plug them in, so you have to have a sufficient supply of batteries—enough for their notorious delays. These small portable, expensive concentrators can be purchased, rented, or in some cases have been (although this is increasingly uncommon) loaned free by one's O2 provider. The Federal Aviation Administration (FAA) must approve each new portable device for use in an airplane, but each airline has the option of adding it or not to the list of those it accepts (or does not accept) for use on board its planes.

- Rules can, and do, change overnight, so check long in advance with your airline.

- If you need to switch planes, be sure to find out who the second carrier is and check its policy also. Don't take the original booking airline's word.

- You can use bottled O2 up to the entrance of the plane and outside of the plane upon reaching your destination. You'll need someone's help to take the O2 with him or her once you board with your concentrator.

- As reimbursement payment to providers of O2 decrease, so will their services. There may be extra fees when assisting travelers.

- Be aware that not all airline personnel are equally trained when it comes to O2-using passengers. Flight attendants are said to have better training regarding our needs than ground personnel. The person who answers your questions on the phone might have yet different training altogether.

- To complicate matters, the airport isn't run by airline personnel! There are the airport employees and security personnel, some of whom don't have a clue about COPD, O2, or reasonable accommodations.

Here are some steps you can take to help ensure a problem-free flight:

1. Call the airline well in advance of your planned travel date to find out its specific O2 policy. Ask about any steps that need to be taken to ensure that the person meeting you with portable O2 tanks (if needed) on the other end of your flight is actually allowed to meet you at the plane. He or she may need to carry a copy of your doctor's prescription, indicating your need for O2 while on the ground, copy of your ticket, note from the Pope...

2. Get the necessary forms from the airline for your doctor to fill out. Your doctor usually faxes these back to the airline. Once you think the process has taken place, give your airline a call to confirm it got all the forms it requires and that they were correctly filled out.

3. If you are running short on battery power, be sure that there is a tank of O2 waiting for you at the gate upon your arrival. The person meeting you might first need to go to the airline's check-in counter, and your airline might need to know in advance that someone will be meeting you. If security officers give the person meeting you a hard time, as has happened, your airline might be able to intervene.

4. There have been instances of airline or security staff not allow-
    ing relatives to meet people at the gate with their O2, thereby
    stranding them at the gate without O2 and/or expecting them
    to walk to the other side of security check points without O2.
    This should be less of a problem now that most travelers will
    be using portable concentrators. They can usually be plugged
    in, to spare or recharge the battery, in the waiting area. Some
    travelers carry power adapters so they can share an occupied
    outlet if it is already in use. If you run into a problem and need
    O2 but can't get it, don't risk your health. If necessary, call
    EMS.

If you find it justified to lodge a complaint, don't just write to
the airline (who will probably make paper planes out of it), also
contact:

> Aviation Consumer Protection Division
> U.S. Department of Transportation
> 400 Seventh St. SW
> Room 4107, C-75
> Washington, D.C. 20590
> http://airconsumer.ost.dot.gov
> (800) 778-4838 (voice)
>
> Federal Aviation Administration
> Consumer Hotline, AOA-20
> 800 Independence Ave. SW
> Washington, D.C. 20591
> (866) 835-5322

Cruise Ship Travel

Although there are special cruises for people with COPD who use
O2, traditional cruise ships should not be ruled out. The larger
ones have a doctor and medical facilities on board; however, each
company has its own policies regarding O2, so check with the
company with whom you are interested in traveling. They vary
widely in how they deal with O2. Some make no special accommodations, while others will make the O2 arrangements for you.
Of course, advanced planning and appropriate documentation
from your doctor are always required.

Whether or not the ADA covers cruise ships that fly foreign flags (most ships) is unclear. Discrimination suits were brought against a few, and some suits were lost, some won, some appealed, reversed, etc., and at least one reached the Supreme Court in 2005. It resulted in a split decision. Nevertheless, ships are becoming more accommodating, especially for wheelchair travelers. Newer ships tend to be designed to be more accommodating than older ships.

There are special cruises available for people on O2. Some are even staffed by a pulmonologist, registered nurse specialists, or by a respiratory therapist (RT) or respiratory therapist technician (RTT). One company, Seapuffers (Pam and Angus Mackenzie, 4 Livingston St., Honeoye Falls, NY 14472, (877) 473-2726 or www.seapuffers.com) provides all the arrangements, including travel with O2 to and from the port of departure. Other resources for cruises and other travel for individuals with disabilities are www.medicaltravel.org and www.cruiseholidays.com. In addition, the American Lung Association (www.lungusa.org) can direct you to special cruises.

Using supplemental O2 when we need it is one of the best things we can do to help our COPD. In addition to O2, keeping active, exercising, and doing whatever else we can to stay healthy are essential. Let's take a look at these other things that can help us to live longer and enjoy the time we have.

Chapter 13

STAYING HEALTHY: NUTRITION, PREVENTING ILLNESSES, AND EXERCISE

If I'd known I was going to live so long, I'd have taken better care of myself.
~ Leon Eldred

People tend to make a distinction between the mind and the body, often suggesting that a problem is either emotionally based or physically based. We know that there are often physical sources for what we think are emotional or psychological problems. For example, abnormal hormone levels, brain abnormalities, and a host of other illnesses affect our emotions. We also know that emotional or psychological problems, including stress, can affect our bodies and change our body's vulnerability, chemistry, and our ability to heal. The truth is that there is no distinct difference between the mind and body; after all, our mind is part of our body, and what affects our body can affect our mind (and vice versa). Staying healthy requires not only attending to our physical health but also our emotional health as well—our bodies and our minds are inseparable partners.

Having pled my case that the mind and body are inseparable, I'm going to stick my foot in my mouth and focus only on our physical health in this chapter. We'll focus on our emotional health later. Being in as good physical health as possible is important, and keeping in good physical health is easier said than done. Besides proper medication, remaining in good shape requires proper nutrition, proper disease prevention, and proper exercise.

Proper Diet

I'm fat and have diabetes. I have no right to tell others how they should eat, but that's not going to stop me! I do know to take multivitamins, stick to complex carbohydrates instead of simple ones, and eat lots of non starchy vegetables and small amounts of lean meat. Some of us have quality-of-food issues (I don't) and some of us have portion control issues (mind your own business)! Some of us have a problem with both. Yet others of us struggle to keep our weight from slipping.

In either case, the best thing we can do for ourselves if we have a weight issue is to consult with a nutritionist and change our eating lifestyle. There are plenty of diets out there to choose from, but it is not just about losing the weight, it is about keeping it off. Many of us find it especially difficult to limit our food intake when on oral prednisone, a corticosteroid. I'd eat the plaster off my walls if I could. One thing I will admit openly, however, is how much my breathing improves when I lose weight. It is, quite frankly, dramatic. Some COPDers think that they cannot lose weight because they can't do enough exercise to increase their metabolism or burn off the calories. I've been told by good sources this is not true. Yes, it helps to exercise, not only because it burns calories but also because it increases your metabolism, but an inability to exercise will not stop you from being able to lose weight. Just do as much as you can—with your doctor's approval, of course!

We COPDers have a unique problem. As the lungs expand in overall size to make up for the loss of lung function, they push everything they can out of the way, and the pressure will, over time, even increase the size of the rib cage, producing the stereotypical "barrel chest" in some people. With this competition for space, a full stomach will interfere with the lungs' ability to fully expand. This makes breathing more difficult, and it is why you might have difficulty breathing after a meal. Smaller and more frequent meals help many of us breathe more easily. This problem affects some people more than others, and for some of us, the very act of eating makes us SOB. I complete all my appointments, chores, or physical efforts before my first meal of the day. After that, I'm shot. Find what works best for you.

Metabolism, in its simplest terms, is breaking down food and O2 (oxygen) into energy and CO2 (carbon dioxide). Digestion requires O2, and because of that some people claim that the extra demand for O2 used for digestion negatively affects our breathing. I don't know if the extra demand for O2 is really great enough to be of concern. We've got to eat so...

There are occasional discussions that carbonated beverages are also not good for us because they contain CO2, which requires extra work for the body to get rid of. I think that the concern with carbonated beverages is more the issue of gas, not the extra CO_2, but that's just my opinion. For the same reason, some doctors will tell us to avoid gassy foods, so stay away from gassy foods unless you find farting—okay, passing gas—somehow entertaining or a way of keeping people from sitting next to you at the casino.

Interestingly, I've also read and would like to believe that because of the extra effort it takes us to breathe, we burn many more calories breathing than people with healthy lungs. Finally, one positive thing about COPD if you are overweight! More need for O_2 with less ability for our lungs to extract it out of the air can be a lethal combination, as it taxes our heart and other organs. Now, don't get jealous of those skinny people either; they have a greater need to be tethered down during windstorms.

General Suggestions

- Eat smaller, more frequent meals.

- Talk to your doctor about multivitamins, particularly those with antioxidants.

- It is well accepted that omega-3 fatty acid is an anti-inflammatory. Good sources are oily fish and flax seed. Beware of their high calorie content, though.

- Eat a diet high in fiber and whole grains. This has been shown to help people with COPD and actually improve lung function.

- I hate to say this, but limit your sodium (salt) intake. Too much salt can lead to water retention (in addition to other medical problems), which will make breathing more difficult. If you are going to use a salt substitute, be aware that some are made of potassium chloride. Check with your doctor to see if it is okay for you to consume potassium chloride and, if so, how much. Too much or too little potassium can be very dangerous.

- Eat your broccoli! Researchers at John Hopkins found that broccoli contains a specific antioxidant that prevents the degradation of a chemical that fights inflammation in the lungs. I first read this, coincidentally, while sipping a cup of broccoli soup, so it must be true!

- Some people say that CoQ10 improves oxygenation, so talk to your doctor to see if he or she recommends it. I've heard mixed things.

- Be sure to get enough calcium, especially if you are on steroids. Calcium also needs vitamin D to help bones absorb calcium. Incidentally, if you take calcium supplements, some types (the ones comprised of calcium carbonate) need to be taken with food in order to be absorbed. I've been told to stay away from the calcium from coral.

- Be sure your intake of vitamin D is adequate, and be sure your doctor checks your vitamin D level. Many North Americans are deficient in vitamin D.

- Avoid cured meats such as ham or bacon that contain nitrites. Nitrites may decrease lung function. Nitrate-free bacon is available in some stores.

- Drink plenty of water and lower your caffeine intake.

I know how to eat well but the hardest part for me comes when I'm not feeling well enough to prepare proper meals. I'll reach for something easy and satisfying. Often, these foods are not the best choices. Preparing and freezing extra meals when you are feeling better is one of the ways to maintain better control during the more difficult times. I also find that preparing dinner in the afternoon, when possible, for reheating later helps me control what I eat.

Exercise

Proper exercise is essential and is one of the limited numbers of things we can do to help our COPD. Discuss any potential exercise program with your doctor before you begin, and ask your doctor about the availability of a pulmonary rehabilitation program, both in terms of availability in your area and insurance coverage. A good medically approved program should not only include the type and frequency of specific exercises, but also the amount of O2 that you should use during those exercises if you are prescribed O2.

A surprising number of COPDers find that gardening brings them both a form of exercise and much satisfaction. Bending over is a major problem for many of us, but it can be reduced if we do "container gardening." A word of caution, however, is that there are some organisms naturally occurring in soil that may cause serious lung infections if we are immune-compromised or our resistance is down. A couple of the infections that seem to pop up once in a while within our COPD community are pseudomonas and aspergillus, but I'm sure there are more. I don't know the degree of risk that is involved, and there is a lot of variation between us COPDers. If you garden or plan to garden, ask your pulmonologist if it is safe for you.

I find grocery stores an ideal place to exercise. I can hold on to the cart (which seems to help me walk farther), rest my O2 tank in the child's seat, rest when I need by stopping and reading labels, and, last but not least, annoy the staff by blocking the aisles when they are trying to stock the shelves. Grocery stores are less crowded early in the morning, are usually climate controlled, and most have bathrooms. You can even track your walking distance and keep a walking progress chart if you desire. A good pedometer might be in order, but check it out before you rely upon it. I tried one once and found it inaccurate for the slow type of walking I was doing. Perhaps somewhere in fine print it stated, "Does not measure waddles," but I returned it for a refund anyway.

Although we are all a bit different in our strides, we can count our strides and, once we measure our strides, determine how far we have walked. You can measure your stride by determining the number of inches in each stride and figuring out how many strides you need to make a mile (5,280 feet), or use the following:

Men average about 2,000 strides per mile.

Women average about 2,400 strides per mile.

Be aware that many consider a mile on a treadmill less strenuous than walking on the ground.

For those with limited mobility, or for those who cannot exercise outside of a wheelchair, there are exercises available that can be done while seated. There are many sources for such information, and they can be found by searching for "wheelchair exercise" or "wheelchair exercise videos" on the Internet. One place you can purchase instructions is www.thewheelchairsite.com. Once again, always check with your physician before starting an exercise program.

Vaccines

Be sure to get your flu shot each year and your pneumonia shot every five years, or as recommended by your physician.

The Importance of Infection Control

A large part of staying healthy is avoiding infections, particularly respiratory infections. Many believe that each infection we get destroys just a bit more of our lungs; perhaps, however, it has more to do with the type of infection. One term that is often used by and around people with COPD is "exacerbation." An exacerbation is a sudden flare-up or increase in symptoms of a chronic illness—in our case, COPD—due to any number of things, such as infections or lung irritations that come from smoke, allergens, fumes, etc.

Signs of infections are generally considered to be a change in sputum color (yellow or green sputum), amount or viscosity (thickness) of sputum, abnormal body temperature, cough or sore throat, aches and pains, fatigue, etc. Infections can be viral, bacterial, or even mold or yeast infections. Antibiotics won't help a viral infection but are sometimes given to reduce the chance of getting a secondary bacterial infection, which is common when the body's resistance is down and mucus membranes are raw and inflamed due to a viral infection or other existing condition that bacteria find attractive. Yeast infections can be made worse with antibiotics, so don't treat yourself with leftover antibiotics without talking to your doctor. Report any unusual symptoms to your doctor even if they don't fit the usual descriptions such as those above. Early treatment can ward off a later disaster.

Preventing infections requires that we limit our contact with germs both at home and when out in public. I've managed almost twenty years with COPD without requiring hospitalization to fight a lung infection. I don't attribute this to either the healthiness of my lungs or my overall health. Instead, I seek antibiotics quickly when needed and, even more important, I am very careful about avoiding contact with germs.

Infection Control

Be careful, very careful, about inviting people in who are sick, whether they are adults or children. If you practice this avoidance successfully, you will step on toes; I promise. Because it is frowned upon to dunk children with sniffles into vats of antiseptic solutions upon their arrival at your home, you must use caution around them. Although professing you are allergic to children might create a tad of mistrust in your family, you need to "educate" their parents (often your own kids) on what they need to do to limit your exposure to sick kids. Never reject a child in front of them, such as shouting, "Get out of here, you diseased little bastard" upon their arrival! Instead, educate their parents on how to explain the situation to the children so that they develop an understanding (as best they can) and so they do not hold themselves responsible for the rejection. Also, never, ever tell kids that you caught something from them; it is like telling them that they hurt you. Be a responsible adult. Blame their parents!

Most adults, even those who are well aware of your COPD, simply don't comprehend the need for you to be careful; they will constantly slip up. Don't expect them to take responsibility to protect you from infectious diseases; if you do, you will be disappointed. It is your responsibility, not theirs. Yes, they'll get annoyed that you keep asking if anyone is sick before a visit, but they'll get over it faster than you'll get over a serious illness. Sadly, you can't take anyone's judgment for granted, and constant questioning is required. Some will offer excuses like, "Oh, it is nothing, it is just smoker's cough." Balderdash!

People can often pass on a bug shortly before or shortly after they begin to show symptoms, so sick people cannot always be identified. Simply being with people will always pose some risk. The only way you can avoid catching a cold or other germ from people is to live on a deserted island by yourself, where, I understand, it is virtually impossible to get cable TV.

If you are not willing to make such a move, there are some things you can do to lessen your chances of catching a bug:

Tips for Avoiding Infections
1. For a start, keeping appropriate distance from people, and knock off all this darn kissing stuff!

2. Walk away from someone sneezing or coughing.

3. Avoid touching your mouth, nose, eyes, or cannula unless your hands are clean. If not through airborne mist from a sneeze or cough, much of your contact with germs will be by way of your hands and then into your body.

4. Wash your hands frequently and well.

5. Do not share towels, utensils, or glasses.

6. Don't drink from the same glass, mug, or straw throughout the day; change it frequently.

7. It only takes a minute to hit the doorknobs with an antibiotic wipe after guests leave.

8. Wash your hands before handling any grocery product just brought into your home. Cashiers are sometimes cited as the second greatest carriers of germs. Actually, they come in second, right after people who provide direct care to others, who claim first prize.

9. Raw and irritated nostrils and mucus membranes are attractive to germs, so frequent saline nasal washes or sprays can be helpful if yours dry out. Seek your doctor's advice on which ones to use and the frequency with which they should be used. Some doctors recommend staying away from nasal washes.

10. Proper humidity throughout the house, room, or simply using an O2 concentrator humidifier is very useful as long as it is properly cleaned.

11. Chronic nasal conditions need to be properly diagnosed and treated by a doctor. Postnasal drip can be a real problem, resulting in a sore throat, and can eventually lead to a lung infection.

12. Also be aware that some medications, such as diuretics, anti-anxiety agents, and other medications, can dry out mucus membranes.

13. Change or disinfect your toothbrush regularly, and more frequently during and after an illness. Ultraviolet light sterilizers are now widely available for some toothbrushes, including electric ones.

14. Rinse and gargle after each nebulizer or inhaler that contains corticosteroids or any other medications that seem to irritate your throat.

15. Change your bed linen often.

16. Avoid places of molds and mildews both at home and outside the home as much as possible.

17. Keep your nebulizer and any other equipment properly cleaned and sanitized. Change your cannula often, and avoid handling and adjusting your nostril piece with dirty hands.

Infection Control When Away from Your Home

There are many things you can do to protect yourself from germs when you leave your home. You can use the same good common sense about avoiding sick people as you do at home by trying to avoid crowds and sick people as much as reasonably possible, something usually hard to do. Eventually, you will pick out a cough or sneeze above the din of noise around you, locate its origin as if you had sonar, and find yourself walking in the opposite direction.

Your hands will come into contact with many germs but your hands usually need to come into contact with your mouth, nose, ears, or eyes in order for them to invade your body, so avoid touching your ear, nose, mouth, or eyes. We often touch them unconsciously. When washing, do an extra good job around the fingertips and nails, and wash for at least 20 seconds in hot, soapy water.

I must warn you not to get too carried away with the numerous recommendations, or worse, become afraid to go out because germs lurk around every corner! My intent is not to frighten you from going out; it is quite the opposite. If you can increase your awareness of how germs are transferred from one person to another, and if you follow at least some of the following tips, you can feel safer when out and enjoying life. And by all means, get out and enjoy your life!

Money

Money, especially paper money, is very dirty; it passes many hands and is often kept in a relatively airtight location with a nice dose of heat and humidity to keep the germs healthy, robust, and anxious to multiply. Wash your hands after handing money.

Car

When getting into your car after an event, store visit, or errand, use a hand sanitizer. Along with wiping your hands, wipe off those things your dirty hands just touched before you cleaned them, such as the steering wheel, door handle, etc.

Restaurants

Don't worry about what comes out of the kitchen; you have no control over that. If you are seated next to or near someone obviously sick, either put a bag over their head or consider moving to a safer locale. Don't be shy. The problem with eating in restaurants, regardless of the type, is not so much your neighbors, but about all the people who ate at your table before you arrived. They left more than a tip for the waiter; they left germs. Having undoubtedly picked you out of the crowd, the germs are waiting patiently and watching your every move, hoping you make a mistake. The germs have set up residence in many locales:

1. Menus (so use a hand cleaner after ordering)

2. Salt and pepper shakers, ketchup bottles, etc.

3. The table and chairs (especially the back of chairs where they are most commonly touched when moving)

4. Lemons in water (ask for no lemons)

There is nothing worse than watching a waitress wipe her nose with her finger and then slip it through the handle of the coffee cup she is bringing to you. Yum, yum! You can hit that with your hand wipe also as well as other things she touched.

If you are eating exclusively with a fork, knife, or spoon, there is less chance of picking up a bug. Just to be polite, I always bring hand wipes along for those with whom I share a meal, but I've given up trying to sell them to the people dining around me at other tables.

Don't accept water with a lemon in it. The waiter grabbed the lemon from a bowl and threw it into your water with his bare hands, so it is kind of like the waiter sticking his finger into your water. Well, isn't it?

Hospitals

Avoid hospitals, nursing homes, or other places sick people congregate. If you can't avoid them, just be aware of everything you touch, including elevator buttons and handrails, then wash or use a hand sanitizer after.

Bathrooms

Public bathrooms have it all backwards. If you think about hand-washing routines in public bathrooms, once you've attended to business, you first turn on the water using levers that everyone else used when their hands were dirty, you then wash your hands, and then again touch the dirty levers before drying, and then you touch the worst place, the doorknob or handle, when exiting the bathroom.

Consider washing and drying your hands and then turning off the water with the hand towel. Use a hand towel, paper towel, or anything you can (including a shirt tail) to open the door when you leave.

Alternately, just use a hand wipe after leaving the bathroom.

There is also controversy over the effectiveness of air hand dryers. Some research concludes that they disperse bacteria within a radius around them and are less effective than using paper towels that also remove surface germs when you use them to dry. If you have a choice, use hand towels, but don't turn a crank to get to get one!

Also be aware of cross contamination of any type of article that you might set on the floor or on the sink in a bathroom. Look for hooks in bathrooms on which to hang your bags to avoid transporting germs to your home.

Casinos

Where can you go that provides entertainment, doesn't require much physical energy or walking, doesn't put on weight, and provides a good distraction? Casinos! These are magnets for people with COPD and are best visited when the crowds are thin. Just imagine the number of people who wiped their nose with their finger prior to hitting all those magical buttons that draw you there. Antibacterial wipes are a necessity. I simply avoid touching my eyes, nose, mouth, or cannula, and sanitize my hands after I lose my allowance. This way I don't have to worry about germs and can push any button I want!

Doctors' Offices

Many doctors' offices have masks and hand sanitizers available. In the United States, we have it backwards. Healthy people use masks to avoid the germs of unhealthy people. Elsewhere in this fine world, sick people often wear them out of concern for the health of others. If your doctor's office doesn't have masks or gel, you might want to suggest it. Ask for an early appointment so there are fewer patients around, and do not show up too early when you know you'll be waiting. Avoid touching the magazines or newspapers in a doctor's office, and I'd suggest sitting as far away from others as you can, especially if they appear ill. However, don't threaten to use pepper spray if they get too close. I found that it attracts too much attention. Bring your own pen to avoid signing in with the pen that sick people use. Even more important than avoiding germs is avoiding them entering your body, so don't touch your eyes, nose, or mouth until after you clean your hands.

Mass Transit

Once again, crowd a bunch of people together, limit the air circulation, and you increase your risk of picking up a bug. Avoid mass transportation if you can, or travel during less congested times. If you live in the city and this is your primary means of transportation, than just accept that mass transportation is part of life and continue to get out and enjoy your life. Once again, avoid touching your mouth, nose, and eyes, and use antibacterial wipes.

Stores

All you need to do is take a look at the checkout staff in the larger grocery stores to see how illnesses are spread. If stores don't provide them, use your own wipes to clean things like grocery cart handles. Remember that the store clerk probably grabbed all of the handles of your bags, so wash your hands after you place them in the car and after unpacking them at home. Also be aware that the pens used to sign our receipt or the keys and buttons that are punched to pay for your products are also full of germs, so bring your own pen and use it not only for signing but also to press all those buttons if you swipe a credit card. Once again, the simplest way is to limit your exposure is to accept that we live in a world of germs and avoid touching your eyes, nose, mouth, or, if you are using 02, your cannula until after you use a hand sanitizer.

Church, Synagogues, Mosques, Temples, and Places of Worship

You can catch some rather faithful germs in places of worship! Praying extra hard will not always replace using antibacterial wipes. It is considered rude to pray out loud that you don't catch the cold from the lady in the next row. Be aware that some of the rituals promoting fellowship and bringing people together can be a bit risky.

Social Events

After a while, you will get used to canceling on people because either you aren't feeling up to the event or you learn of someone ill who plans on attending the event. It will often be at the last minute and will annoy others. There is no escaping this. Choose your events carefully, and don't let family or friends dictate what is safe for you. It is your responsibility. You might lose friends along the way and people might give up on inviting you. That's why there are casinos.

Even the best of practices cannot protect us from all illnesses and exacerbations. If you follow some of the above tips, they should be fewer and further apart. However, when they do occur, you should be prepared to handle illnesses, emergencies, and even be prepared in the event that you need to be hospitalized. There are many things you can do to be prepared. You will be rewarded for being well prepared; you'll get faster, more appropriate medical attention, eliminate some of the stress involved, and take some burden from those people upon whom you rely to help when such events occur.

Chapter 14

EMERGENCIES, HOSPITALIZATIONS,VENTILA-

TORS, AND ADVOCACY

A hospital is no place to be sick.
~ *Redd Foxx*

An ounce of prevention…ah, you know the rest! Yup, it holds true here, too. If you haven't successfully avoided catching a bug, contact your doctor as soon as you can. Also contact your doctor if you are having greater breathing problems than you are accustomed to having or notice changes to your sputum. Because some of us have frequent breathing problems, talk to your doctor early in your relationship about when to call him or her or head off to an ER. Many doctors will provide you with an emergency antibiotic to use when symptoms of an infection occur, such as fever or discolored sputum. They will tell you when and only when to use it. Indiscriminate use of medications, including antibiotics, is harmful. Your doctor might need to know you fairly well before giving you emergency antibiotics. Others want to be called first, and only then will they decide if you need an antibiotic. Whether or not your doctor gives you an emergency antibiotic is not a fair way to judge a doctor, so just accept his or her policy and call on weekends. Why weekends? Well, we all know that we usually get sick on weekends, holidays, or when pharmacies are closed! Germs, I understand, keep calendars and look forward to the holidays as much as we do. It is their busy season, too, after all, and the holiday get-to-gethers provide them with all the social contact they need to spread their special form of cheer.

Summoning Emergency Help
There are many home emergency monitoring devices available, and people who are vulnerable shouldn't have to wait for an emergency to be convinced of their merits. Home monitoring systems are medical alert devices that are monitored 24 hours a day for a monthly or yearly fee for the service. You wear a wireless device around your

neck, key chain, watch, or as a bracelet, and press the call button if you need help, often through a small speaker system. The service will respond according to the instructions you gave when you set up the service.

You may also want to consider leaving a key in a security lock box near your door in order for help to gain access. Your monitoring company can give EMS the code. It is also a way for friends or relatives to check on you in the event you do not answer your phone or door. Avoid leaving your key under your front mat or under the ceramic frog just to the right of your door.

Cell Phones

Not only are cell phones useful when you are out of your home, they can be useful within your home. If you have an emergency and are unable to move about and call for help, you can phone someone—even if they live in the same house but cannot hear you! Just be sure to carry it around with you, including into the bathroom.

Emergency Medical Information: Medical Alert Bracelets, Necklace Tags, and Medical Fact Sheets

There are many types of medical alert bracelets and necklace tags that are available on which emergency information can be engraved. Some have medical cards that come with them that can be kept in your wallet, or that instruct the rescuer on how to access medical information you have entered into the company's databank. They are great as long as you remember to wear them and pay the hefty price to update them (the bracelets, that is) when changes occur to your medications (if listed on the bracelet). Alternatively, emergency medical information can be stored on a flash drive that snaps into computers and which, because it is small, can be attached to your keychain. It is easy to update, and all the ER has to do is plug it in to access your medical records.

Cell phones are also a place EMS workers *sometimes* check for emergency information if they cannot find the information elsewhere. However they are more likely to stabilize you and get you to a hospital rather than playing with your cell phone. Although storing emergency information in your phone under ICE (In Case of Emergency) started as a rumor, the rumor became so popular that it actually caught on and people are doing it!

When to Seek Emergency Help

Of course, most people don't want to call their doctors or head off to the emergency room, but procrastination is not smart. If you need help, get it. It is your job. Don't hesitate calling an ambulance if needed. If you are not dressed and are too SOB to get dressed, don't worry about it, they'll take care of that, your house keys, and whatever else is needed. Remember, they do that for a living! EMS can start treatment long before you would get treatment if you got yourself to an emergency room. Because of the pervasiveness of our disease, ERs are usually well equipped and prepared to handle us COPDers. I say "usually" because there are glaring exceptions.

Be Prepared

Long before you even get to the point of calling an ambulance, you need to prepare for the possibility. Everyone should have three, maybe four things prepared in advance:

1. A Vital Information Sheet (also referred to as a "File of Life") consisting of all of your pertinent medical information printed out neatly on paper, as listed in the chapter on doctors. Just be sure to keep your list updated! When the time comes for them to collect information from you, it is much more pleasant to breathe than have to respond to their many necessary questions. You may want to carry a copy of this information with you everywhere you go, give a copy to a friend, and leave a copy on your refrigerator door.

2. Pack a hospital bag for someone to grab on your behalf in case you happen to be admitted to a hospital. Asking someone to put one together after you are admitted is an unnecessary burden, and you know as well as I do that they will screw up your instructions!

3. Have an advocate. Plan in advance for someone to accompany you to the hospital or meet you there. Emergency rooms and hospitals are dangerous places and no place for decent sick people to have to advocate for their own care if they are so sick that they need to be in an ER!

4. Consider a riding crop. Taking a riding crop along with you to a hospital is optional; however it does have advantages. It can be used to threaten sick medical personnel should they either sneeze on you or not wash their hands properly. Plan to use it defensively only. Hide it if you hear them paging a psychiatrist.

Emergency Rooms

Emergency rooms are hard on everyone—staff and patients alike. Time moves slowly, comfort is not a necessity, and your care is not based exclusively upon your needs. Your care is also based upon what else is happening in the ER at the time you are there. If you are a walk-in, you can expect to wait. If you are desperate and have a large asthmatic component, mention the asthma attack; it should get you in more quickly. If you arrive by ambulance, you'll get faster attention but might have to make up for the initial speed later. As long as you are stabilized, that's okay. Be patient. Be aware that they are not there to treat your overall condition; they are there to treat the emergency so that you can be safely released for follow-up by your own doctor.

Hospitalizations

Hospitals are dangerous. Stay away from them. They are full of sick people, resistant germs, unsanitary conditions, and overworked medical staff! Infection control is a major problem in most hospitals.

It is the job of medical workers to protect both us and them, and that's a big assignment. One of the biggest problems in infection control is that some medical staff often seem to better remember to take measures to protect themselves rather than their patients. Yes, they will wear gloves to protect themselves from germs, but in some cases they continue to touch people and objects with those same dirty gloves. Although infection control practices might have improved over the years, it has not gotten to the point where you can let down your guard. Many hospitals are having serious problems with the transmission of antibiotic-resistant organisms. Problems are common enough to warrant warning you to both maintain your vigilance and speak up when and if necessary. When you have the thought, "Maybe I should say something," don't ponder it, speak up! If you feel later that you were "out of place," you can always apologize.

Do not let any medical personnel touch you or treat you unless they have washed or sanitized their hands. It is real hard to speak up at times and "correct" a nurse or doctor, but one case of a resistant infection, now more common than ever in hospitals, can be worse than the illness for which you were admitted. I speak from personal experience.

The number of medication administration errors in hospitals is often cited as being quite high and frightening. If you can, keep track of what you are taking, especially if there are changes. For this, having an "advocate," a trusted friend or family member on hand, staying on top of things is most valuable. Let this person know you would like him or her to be assertive on your behalf yet respectful of hospital staff.

Comfort is very important for us but is not on the priority list in most hospitals. Having family and friends around to help you adjust and change positions is almost expected and always appreciated. Frankly, nursing staffs are usually overworked and unable to keep up with anything more than the most important needs.

Some people don't get it. They think hospitalizations are occasions to demonstrate love and support, and so they show up in droves, sometimes waiting in the main reception area for other visitors to leave so they can use their "pass" to go up to visit you. If you don't keep these annoying people away for your own sake, please keep them away for the well-being of your roommate!

If you can afford it, consider private duty nursing for a day or so if needed, especially after surgery or a serious illness. Hospitals have a list of nurses available who are approved by, and familiar with, the hospital. Hospitals have all the information needed to arrange private duty nursing, but you must plan in advance.

Do not be a pest or act like you are in an expensive luxury hotel—they'll just keep your bedpan in the refrigerator to get even with you. Treating hospital staff with kindness and a smile will get you much further than being a grumpy or angry patient. Nurses chose their profession not only because they enjoy forcibly removing your hair with adhesive bandages, they also want to help people on occasion! It is human nature that they enjoy taking care of pleasant patients and don't enjoy taking care of crabby ones.

If you are having problems and your polite approach hasn't worked, you can ask to speak to the "patient advocate." A patient advocate can intervene for you if your concern is serious enough and appropriate.

Hospitals commonly fall short of adequate discharge plans and, according to many, push patients out too fast. Frankly, if they feel that you have someone who will "take care of you" at home, they feel safer and are willing to take greater risks. Further, Medicare has very strict admission and discharge criteria that they must stick to in order to ensure reimbursement. People will sometimes be discharged with plans for home care, but it may take days before the home care agency gets someone in to evaluate your needs. Warn your advocate to do what he or she can to ensure a smooth transition.

Sometimes you are no longer in need of hospitalization but you are not quite ready to be at home either. Inpatient rehabilitation centers can often bridge the gap. Sometimes you, the patient, need to be the first one to mention this possibility. Don't hesitate to ask.

Remember that there is a social work or case management department in your hospital and that it specializes in putting the pieces together, arranging services and creating links that could greatly benefit you. The social workers are sometimes referred to as case managers. If you need to apply for a public program such as Welfare or Medicaid, for example, find out if they can apply for you while you are still at the hospital.

The type of aftercare and assistance you can receive at home depends on your insurance, your state, and your age. If you have private insurance, you need to familiarize yourself with the company's policy. If you have Medicare, you are entitled to some home health care, such as nursing visits and physical and occupational therapy. Some states expand the service to include transportation, personal assistance with bathing, shopping, etc., either through Medicare, state services, or even local services. Some services are for people who are disabled, and others services for people who meet age requirements. Your social worker at the hospital will have all the information and contacts you need and can even set things up if you give him or her enough time.

Ventilators and Intubation

Nothing seems to scare us more than the thought of requiring hospitalization and then being put on a ventilator when in a hospital. This represents, at least for some of us, total lack of control. Those of us with COPD know that our chance of requiring assistance to breathe when seriously ill is greater than the average person's. Most of us are terrified at the prospect of being on a ventilator. I have found that knowing more about it has eased my fears; so if you are trembling, you can calm down and not be afraid to read on.

Terminology Time

It is terminology time, but there aren't many terms, so this will go quickly. The terms "respirators" and "ventilators," although referring to different things, are often used interchangeably by nonmedical people. Those in the medical field know that we use them interchangeably (and incorrectly) and therefore they have often given up trying to correct us when we use the wrong term. Technically, ventilators assist or replace spontaneous breathing (which is the topic here), and respirators, on the other hand, are things, usually masks that we wear, to clean the air of pollutants such as gasses, fumes, and filters. You can also see why the terms are easily confused. We are going to talk about ventilators only.

Types of Ventilators

There are two types of ventilators; one type is the "invasive" type because it requires a tube be put into an individual's airway. The other type is "noninvasive" because it uses a tight-fitting mask instead of a tube and works exclusively through air pressure. I must warn you that many people, including professionals, do not usually refer to this passive type as a ventilator. When they talk about "ventilators," they usually mean the invasive type.

You might hear the word "vented," as in, "Joan was vented." That usually means she was hooked up to a ventilator, the "invasive type." By "hook up," people are usually referring to a tube being inserted into the airway and down into the lungs through which air (O2 enriched or not) can flow in and out of the lungs from the ventilator that creates the needed pressure to inflate and deflate the lungs. Putting this tube in is called "intubation," or, if used as a verb, "Joan was intubated." Conversely, "extubation" means removing the tube.

The noninvasive type of ventilator is often simply referred to as a BiPAP machine; however, not commonly known is that the word "BiPAP" is a brand name! The correct term for this noninvasive ventilator is "bi-level noninvasive ventilator." This type of ventilator creates air pressure to inflate and deflate the lungs. Instead of a tube into the airway, the bi-level noninvasive machines allow the user to wear a close-fitting face mask (of which there are many types and varieties). They are small units and can be used at home, usually only at night during sleep. They assist rather than takes over your breathing. That's the end of the terminology. Now admit out loud that it wasn't bad!

What It Is Like to Be Vented

The situation most of us fear—being ventilated while ill—is often a bit different than we imagine (if it has crossed our mind). When intubation is needed, we are often so ill or are medicated to the point of not being very aware of the procedure. We might remain heavily medicated once intubated, or we might be fully conscious; this all depends on the particulars of the person, the nature of the problem, type of tube, and the treatment plan. Often, we may start off heavily medicated and then have the medication slowly withdrawn.

Length and Process

How long you stay ventilated depends on the severity of your exacerbation or illness and the underlying state of your lungs and other vital organs, especially your heart and kidneys. Most people with an acute COPD exacerbation are only ventilated for two to four days. Because this is no picnic, you will be given sedating and pain medications. When you are ventilated, you will probably be in an intensive care unit at the hospital because your vital signs and blood gases need to be monitored very closely. You will be sedated and dependent on the nurses to maintain your bodily functions. Usually, at least once each day, the sedation will be stopped and your breathing will be tested to see if your lungs are strong enough to breathe on your own. This is called a "spontaneous breathing trial." If you pass, they remove the breathing tube and dance the merengue around your bed to celebrate. You may need to be sedated once again when you see the hospital bill.

Once off of the ventilator, our vocal cords might need time to recover, and they might be hoarse for a while. During this period, when we are least able to verbally defend ourselves, friends and relatives will try to make up all kinds of stories about how your behavior was inappropriate, which you cannot recall. They'll give vivid descriptions of all the foul language that you used—none of which, of course, you can recall. Some people have no memory of being on a ventilator, while others have only vague memories. Still others have fairly good recall.

Our Unique Situation

Because we have a lung disease, we need to perhaps approach the discussion of whether or not to be intubated (put on a ventilator) a bit differently than most people. Because of our COPD, we may need to be on a ventilator temporarily when fighting an infection or other disease, or simply to compensate for our lousy lungs when recovering from an illness or surgery. Our chance of needing help from a ventilator during an illness (particularly one that affects the lungs) is greater than average. Be absolutely sure that you, your family, and your health care proxy understand the difference between using a ventilator as a support through an illness as opposed to being on a ventilator when there is little, if any, chance of recovery. They are two very different issues, and confusion is common!

Fear of Long-Term Ventilation
We sometimes react very negatively to the idea of ventilators because of the imagined risk of having to remain on one indefinitely. We start to think about such things as when to "pull the plug." Situations such as these are usually very different than situations requiring a vent to help get us through an illness. Nevertheless, there are things you can do to ensure you are not put on a ventilator indefinitely.

Advanced Planning for Your Medical Care
There are a few very important things you can do to insure your medical care is the type that you desire. It is best to discuss these with a local attorney because state laws sometimes differ. Although they are discussed more fully in the chapter called "Put it In Writing," they are:

Advanced Directives
Advanced directives are written instructions that specify what health care you want or do not want if you are sick or injured. You can make your decisions regarding care and treatment choices now (in writing) and/or name someone to make those decisions for you (see "Health Care Power of Attorney" below).

Living Will
A living will is a formal document that provides instructions, but is different from other advanced directives in that it deals with the issue of life support (food, water, ventilator, etc.) when you are deemed to be in a terminal condition by your doctor and are not able to speak for yourself.

DNR Orders (Do Not Resuscitate)

Some people don't complete the other more detailed directives described above that are covered in a living will and just focus on one of the big ones, the DNR (do not resuscitate) order. Hospitals also push this. If you need to be resuscitated (revived from unconsciousness or possible impending death), the procedure is something that has to be done immediately, and medical personnel do not have time to start asking questions or looking through files. Unless you have a DNR order, you will be revived.

Organ Donation

You can decide now if you want your organs donated to others or your body to science.

Health Care Power of Attorney

A power of attorney authorizes someone you designate to make decisions for you. There are different types. One, the financial power of attorney, designates a person as having the power or authorization to handle your nonmedical affairs, such as property and finances. The second type, the type we are more concerned with here, is the health care power of attorney (also known as health care proxy). This allows an appointed individual to make medical decisions when you are not able to do so yourself—a status determined by your physician. How this works depends upon the laws of your particular state. You can specify the types of decisions they can make and impose any limits that you want.

Discuss Your Plans

You might also want to discuss your plans with your physician prior to formalizing them; your doctor might bring up some interesting points you ordinarily might not consider and answer any questions you might have. Because doctors have a huge patient load, it is not reasonable to assume they will remember the finer details of your discussions or even be able to locate copies of the paperwork you gave them. In the event it is needed, your doctor will most likely turn to your next of kin for assistance in locating any required documentation.

Make Copies

Be sure to make many copies of all of your paperwork and to include a copy that is kept in a safe place. Give copies to those named in the documents involved in your care, and have copies on hand to take to your doctor and hospital.

There is no doubt that during the course of a serious illness, especially if it includes a hospital stay, you will become all too familiar with some of the medical equipment used within a hospital setting. There is also equipment that is frequently used within one's own home. You might want to become at least familiar with some of the most common ones, because you will be more comfortable if you know what they are, how they are used, and what to expect when they are used.

Chapter 15

MEDICAL EQUIPMENT, ADAPTIVE EQUIPMENT, AND USEFUL AIDES

One difference between a man and a machine is that a machine is quiet when well oiled.
~ *Anonymous*

There are a few mechanical things out there to make our lives easier, and it is useful to be aware they exist in case we need them. Some of these items can be purchased without a prescription and some require one. If they are covered by your insurance company, you will always need a prescription. If they are prescription items, related to a prescription item, or recommended by your doctor, you can also talk to your tax advisor about taking your out-of-pocket costs off of your taxes as a medical expense.

Before you get durable medical equipment that is covered by Medicare, be sure the company is a "Medicare participating provider." This means that the seller agrees with Medicare to charge a set amount for the piece of equipment, and not anything more. Medicare usually pays 80% of the approved amount, with you or your insurance company paying the remaining 20% of that approved amount. If the seller is not a Medicare participating provider, it can charge what it wants, and you pay the difference between what Medicare pays and what it charges. To find out if Medicare pays for a particular piece of equipment and the names of companies that are Medicare participating providers in your area, visit www.medicare.gov or talk to your doctor.

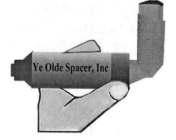

Ye Olde Spacer, Inc

Spacer

Spacers
Spacers are simple tubes (or other shapes) that you use with a MDI (metered dose inhaler). You insert your inhaler into one end of the tube, activate your MDI, and inhale

the mist from the opposite end of the tube. Its purpose is to disperse the medication into a mist before you inhale it to improve the delivery of the medication to your lungs where you need it. It can sometimes compensate for poor technique when using an inhaler. Don't be surprised if your doctor doesn't recommend one. They are more commonly used for asthma than for COPD, although many of us have an asthmatic component to our COPD, and may not work well with the newer inhalers.

Nebulizers

Nebulizers are an alternative to using an MDI (metered dose inhaler, but more commonly referred to as just an inhaler). When your inhalers no longer seem to be as effective as they used to, or during an illness, you will be introduced to the nebulizer. Nebulizers are small electric or battery-powered machines that take liquid medication, usually diluted in a saline solution and in premeasured plastic vials (or ampoules), and turn the solution into a fine mist, which you inhale though a mouthpiece or mask. Chances are that if you use O2, your provider might also carry nebulizers and medications for the nebulizer.

Most people agree that nebulizers are more effective than inhalers, but they are far less convenient. There are many brands and models from which to choose. If you get one through your insurance company, you will probably not be given a choice, and it will be a cheap one. There are many that can easily fit in a handbag, fanny pack, or even large pocket, and that operate

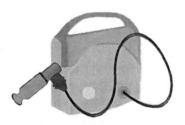

Nebulizer

on regular house current, your car battery (with an adapter), or batteries. I keep a portable one in my car and my regular one plugged in at home. If I'm out for any length of time and in someone else's car, I still take my portable nebulizer with me. It is also good to have a battery battery-powered one in case of power failure.

There are two types of nebulizers, and they differ in the way in which the medication is turned to mist. The most widely used and most economical are those that use compressed air to create a mist from the liquid. The second type doesn't use forced air but instead uses ultrasound to break the liquid into a fine mist, a mist supposedly finer than the mist from compressed air. The purported advantage is that the finer mist gets deeper into the lungs. Although popular (and more expensive), they require elaborate cleaning, and some of them do not work with at least one of the medications often used in a nebulizer, budesonide (e.g., brand Pulmicort), because budesonide is too thick. Incidentally, if you are stuck without electricity and have a continuous flow O2 tank, you might be able to use a high flow setting to create enough pressure to force O2 through the tube to your nebulizer cup.

Most, if not all, nebulizers have filters; some are washable and some need to be replaced. Providers tend to ignore this completely, so you have to go out of your way to get them.

Pulse Oximeters

A pulse oximeter is a small device with a clip that fits on one's finger and measures one's pulse as well as the level of O2 in one's blood. There is a full explanation of this device in the chapter on O2. If you skipped that chapter, hang your head low, apologize, and go back and read it. I'll wait for you here. Don't dawdle!

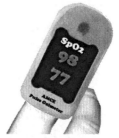

Pulse Oximeter

Lung Exercisers

There are a few mechanisms available for respiratory training. These contraptions are usually a form of a tube that you breathe into and out from that have some resistance. The idea is that you strengthen your respiratory muscles and/or help move residual air out of your lungs by using one of these. There are specific ones that are used after surgery to get the lungs working better. Others on the market work on both the inhalation and exhalation and have adjustable levels of resistance. They are sold on the Internet specifically for people with COPD as well as for athletes to build up their stamina. Not dissimilar, the notion that playing the harmonica or blowing up balloons is similarly helpful. However, I've heard

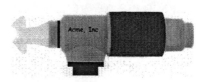

**Resistance
Lung Exerciser**

occasional warnings from people whose doctors told them *absolutely not* to blow up balloons or use any of these devices because doing so can be dangerous if too much force is used! Once again, check with your doctor before you use one of these.

Airway Clearance Devices

There are a number of vests and similar in-struments that are used to vibrate or help loosen mucus. They are used especially for people with bronchiectasis or cystic fi-brosis. The vests can be extremely pricey. There are also small instruments that you breathe through that vibrate or (called "flutter valves") or flutes to help break up mucus and secretions. The brand name of one, Acapella, seems to be the most common. They are available for under $100. These are es-tablished medical devices, so ask your doctor or a respiratory thera-pist about them if you think you need one.

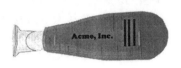

Vibrator

Continuous Positive Airway Pressure Machines (CPAP) and Bi-Level Non-Invasive Ventilators (commonly referred to as BiPAP machines, but BiPAP is a brand name)

A surprising large number of peo-ple with COPD also have sleep ap-nea, a condition in which you stop breathing when sleeping. For more about sleep apnea, see the chapter on common secondary illnesses. Both CPAP (continuous positive air-way pressure) and BIPAP (bi-level positive airway pressure) machines are used by people with sleep ap-

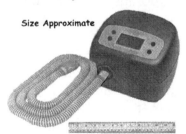

Size Approximate

CPAP/BiPap Machine

nea and are covered by most insurance companies. Briefly, CPAP ma-chines produce air pressure to keep your breathing passages open during sleep. A mask or nose piece is connected to the unit though a hose. A bi-level positive airway pressure machine has the pressure that the CPAP has, but it also reverses the pressure to assist exhal-ing. It is also considered a passive respirator in that it assists rather than takes over breathing. These are sometimes used for people who retain too much CO_2, especially when acutely ill with a COPD exacerbation.

Walkers and Rollators

Once again, these have little to do with COPD but are commonly used. There are many types of walkers that are available that bear some of your weight and help to steady you. A much more popular variation of a walker is the "rollator." Rollators are like sturdy collapsible walkers on wheels, often with a basket for storage of essentials (such as your gin bottle) and a place to sit, which is why they are so popular. They even come with hand breaks. They are available in many different designs, weights, and colors. COPDers often rest their O2 tank in the optional basket and are able to sit on them when tired. They are even available for extra-large people. If you are thinking of purchasing one, double check the total width of the rollator and compare it with some of the doorways inside of your home. They may be a bit too wide to make it through some doors even though they should have no problem with the larger entrance and exit doors.

Collapsible Grocery Carts

Although they don't provide the support of a walker or rollator, they can make life a bit easier. Used primarily to haul or carry things, including groceries and O2, they are collapsible and can fit into a car trunk. There are a few models that have pivoting front wheels that make them able to turn on a dime and are much better than the ones with fixed front wheels. The ones with four pivoting wheels are somewhat harder to find but worth the look.

Wheelchairs

Wheelchairs can get you places that you can't get to on your own. The big disadvantage of having one is that its availability might have the effect of discouraging you from trying to move around on your own, thereby reducing the exercise you need to maintain your health. There are many brands and types available; some are just for "transport" (lightweight and small wheels) and some are for longer-term use. If you are considering an electric wheelchair, also think ahead about ramps, lifts, and even proper vehicles to transport you in one.

Electric Scooters

For use both within and outside the home, electric scooters are an alternative to wheelchairs but are generally not used for sitting for the length of time that wheelchairs are designed to be used. Some come with optional O2 holders. Medicare and other insurance cover them if medically necessary and if needed to get around inside your home.

Shower Stool or Shower Chairs

Shower chairs are a blessing, especially when used together with a handheld shower head. Try to get a metal rather than a plastic handheld shower head, because they are less likely to harbor strange bacteria which, when airborne, have the potential to cause serious lung infections. There are also many other bath-related devices available to make showering easier, including sponges on a stick, battery-powered things that swirl, etc.

While on the subject, take a look around your bathroom to see if there are enough hand bars and rails available to help you shower and use the facilities safely. There are many adaptive devices that help you enter and exit the shower safely. You can always do an Internet search for "handicap shower equipment," "disability bathing devices," and such similar searches. You'll be surprised by what is out there and may come up with a list of things you never knew you needed!

Beds

Hospital beds, if prescribed, are covered by most insurance companies. You usually get the basic (cheap) model, but you may want to look around at some of the better ones. Some are more comfortable than others, and some, in addition to being able to raise the head and feet, also have the ability to raise and lower the whole bed. Sleeping with a raised head helps many people with COPD sleep better. It is also often also prescribed for people with acid reflux disease.

Smoke Masks

If you live in an apartment building or in an area that may require some walking to get away from smoke, you might consider purchasing a smoke mask.

Cold Air Masks

There are a few brands of heat retaining face masks that can be useful in cold weather. They warm the air you inhale by trapping some of the heat and humidity when you exhale. The trapped heat and humidity is used to warm and humidify your next breath.

Other Adaptive Living Aids

There are a large number of adaptive aids available to make it easier for you to do a number of things. One of my favorites is the pincher-grabber-extend-an-arm-thing. A quick look at any catalogue or adaptive aids Web site will reveal many other useful tools. If you can afford it, think big and have a stair lift or elevator put in!

Beyond Equipment

You can have every piece of equipment available and still have breathing problems. Fortunately, for some but not all of us, we might be candidates for surgical intervention. New techniques are being developed to alter the diseased portions of the lungs. Doing so has benefited many people, me being one of them. It is important to be aware of what surgical procedures are available. If interested in surgery, you might want to talk to your doctor about whether you might benefit or are a good candidate for one of the forms of surgery.

Chapter 16

SURGICAL APPROACHES AND TRANSPLANTS

By trying we can easily learn to endure adversity—another man's, I mean.
~ *Mark Twain*

One of the happiest days of my life was the day I received the news that I met the acceptance criteria for lung reduction, a surgery that held the promise of helping my breathing. The mere thought of being able to wake up one day and breathe better was cause to rejoice. I had my surgery in 1994. It was a great success!

What I had was an LVRS (lung volume reduction surgery), one of the four surgical approaches for treatment of COPD. The first two types I'll describe, bullectomies and LVRS, are closely related. The third type, airway bypass, is an alternative to the major surgery described above but achieves much the same result. Finally, I'll briefly explain the fourth type, lung transplant.

Bullectomies
This is the oldest approach and is the surgical removal of inflated bullae, or large distended air sacs in the lungs. It usually involves the removal of one or more of these large air sacs that take up room and therefore impede the healthier parts of the lungs from expanding and working to their top capacity. I don't hear of this being done often but have read that candidates for this surgery are usually younger and have very discernable and large bullae.

Lung Volume Reduction Surgery (LVRS)
LVRS is similar to bullectomies in that hyper inflated bullae (large air sacs) are removed, but rather than just removing a limited number of larger bullae as in a bullectomy, small sections of the lungs are removed. The section of the lungs removed usually contains numerous smaller hyper inflated bullae. This procedure can now be done using video-assisted thoracoscopic surgery (VATS). This allows surgeons to operate through small incisions using high-tech electronic computers

and imaging. They are even making progress on a nonsurgical technique that uses a bronchoscope to get to the diseased areas and dissolve them with a gel or insert stents. My surgeon didn't have this sophisticated technology back when I had my lung reduction. I think I heard him ask for his "Black and Decker Cordless" shortly before I "went under."

Candidates for this surgery are usually those with discernable damage to the upper lobes of their lungs, something often characteristic of smokers. You must meet specific eligibility criteria for this surgery, and Medicare has only approved a few centers to perform lung reductions. You need to be referred to one of these centers by your doctor.

Airway Bypass
There are also a variety of new devices and surgical approaches being investigated that no doubt will soon be available to deal with the hyper inflated bullae (large air sacs) by inserting "stents" or other devices such as valves that allow trapped air to get out of specific sections of the lungs. Think of a stent as a tiny straw. If you place one in an otherwise collapsing airway, it will help the air flow. It works according to the same principal as lung reduction does, but instead of removing the large air sacs, it allows them to deflate so that healthier lung tissue can use the space.

Lung Transplants
Lung transplants are probably the closest thing to a cure for COPD. After lung transplants, patients are usually able to engage in physical activities typical for their age. That is nothing less than amazing! Both single and double lung transplants are available; however, there is usually a long waiting list, usually around two years—give or take a couple of years. Donors are not matched on the first-come, first-served basis, however. There is a great deal of testing done before getting on a transplant list to ensure you are sick enough to need one, yet healthy enough to undergo the transplant.

People often complain about the number of medications that must be taken daily for the rest of your life if you have a transplant. I added them up; they are fewer than I now take. However, it is the type of drugs that must be taken that can be a problem. They include medications to suppress your immune system, as well as antibacterials, antifungals, and antivirals to offset the suppressed immune system. They take their toll. Basically, it is often said that you exchange one disease (COPD) for another because of the transplant.

Many people find the survival rate for lung transplant patients discouraging. Currently, about 80% survive one year, 60% survive three years and just over 40% for five years; however, there is reason to believe that these numbers will be increasing as newer medications and procedures are developed.

I recently wrote to eleven COPDers who had lung transplants, and they answered a bunch of my questions. All eleven were extremely enthusiastic, never had a moment of regret, and all would do it again in a second. Those who didn't live long enough to answer my questions might have had a different opinion.

The Second Wind Lung Transplant Association (www.2ndwind. org or 888-855-9463) is the primary source for information on lung transplants.

In any case, if you are interested in the possibility of a lung transplant, the first step is to talk to your pulmonologist to determine whether he or she thinks you are a candidate. If your doctor thinks you are eligible, you will undergo further comprehensive testing. The decision to have a lung transplant, if approved, is a very difficult one.

Whether or not you are fortunate enough to have surgery, or even be a candidate for surgery, you still run the risk of acquiring one of the illnesses that are related to COPD. Having COPD can lead to other medical problems, so it is wise to know what they are so you can do your best to protect yourself from them.

Chapter 17

COMMON SECONDARY MEDICAL PROBLEMS WITH COPD

The greater the obstacle, the more glory in overcoming it.
~ Moliere

If dealing with COPD isn't enough, we are often hit with other illnesses or medical conditions as well—some directly associated with COPD, some just more common with COPD, and some that have nothing to do with COPD. They all take their toll, both physically and emotionally. Although we should be thankful that we have survived long enough to get another illness, it is not something we tend to celebrate. Knowing a bit about other common secondary medical problems might help us in two ways: first to encourage (or scare us) into staying as healthy as we can to prevent them; and second, to recognize them early in their development so we can seek timely medical attention.

Surgery
Before we even talk about other illness, you are hereby warned to avoid any illness or disease that may require surgery using general anesthesia. As COPD progresses, the risks involved in having surgery with anesthesia increases because the lungs become more compromised. Of course, the degree of risk of any surgery has everything to do with the specific type of surgery that is needed, status of the individual's lungs, and other factors. The closer the surgical site is to your lungs, the more likely it is to interfere with your breathing. Toe surgery is better than gall bladder surgery!

Flu and Pneumonia
The flu can not only make you feel miserable, it can be much more serious for those of us with COPD. Contact your doctor if you have any symptoms such as fever, increased SOB, cough, chest pain, or changes in sputum, such as thickening, amount, or color.

Pneumonia is extremely dangerous for those of us with COPD and can even be life threatening. There are many different types, and they can be caused by viruses, bacteria, and even fungi. The symptoms of cough, fever, chest pain, and SOB make it hard for us to differentiate it from bronchitis or other illnesses; however, your doctor must absolutely be called if you have any symptoms. A pneumonia vaccine covers about one-third of the known bacteria that cause pneumonia, but does not cover the viral or fungal types. Many doctors administer the vaccine to people with COPD about every five years, although the frequency is up to the each physician.

There is also something called "aspiration pneumonia." Aspiration pneumonia develops when foreign material enters the lungs, i.e., food, nasal secretions, particles of matter from acid reflux, or even fumes. This is why you should take acid reflux (also known as GERD—gastro esophageal reflux disease) seriously and discuss proper treatment with your doctor.

Nodules

All too often, CAT scans will detect nodules, unusual growths, or suspicious spots in the lungs. It is important to be aware that nodules are somewhat common in ex-smokers older than the age of 50. Whereas the next step might logically be to perform a biopsy of a nodule, this is often not done for people with COPD for fear that the lung will collapse. It is up to your doctor(s) to determine the best course of action. Although we might be frightened that they are cancer, because some are, the nodules may simply be due to scar tissue from lung infections and other causes. Your doctor will want to monitor your condition and compare CAT scans periodically. If you have nodules, you might also ask for a sputum culture to be done if your doctor doesn't bring it up first. I had a type of infection (a serious one) that formed nodules that was discovered through a sputum culture. I was the one who initiated the discussion of performing a sputum culture.

Heart Problems

CAD (Coronary Artery Disease)

This is a condition in which plaque builds up inside the coronary arteries, the arteries that supply your heart with O2-rich blood. This is the leading killer among smokers. Your risks decline quickly once you give up smoking, but this, when combined with COPD, is a common cause of death for those of us with COPD.

CHF (Congestive Heart Failure)
COPD puts a lot of stress on the heart and circulatory system. As a direct consequence to diminished lung functioning, the heart tries to compensate for the lack of O2 and does more work than it was designed to do. This can result in a few different heart conditions, to include enlargement of the heart (or parts of the heart), fluid retention, etc. Be aware that any edema (which means swelling) of the legs, ankles, or abdomen should result in a call to your doctor. Fluid may also accumulate in the lungs, which will lead to a shortness of breath, being able to breathe only in certain positions, and even gasping for breath during the night. As some of the breathing symptoms of CHF are similar to symptoms of COPD, it is important that you report all of your symptoms or changes in your symptoms immediately to your doctor.

Cor Pulmonale
Cor pumonale is the failure or significant changes in the right ventricle of the heart that pumps blood to the lungs. It is caused by pulmonary hypertension.

Pulmonary Hypertension
Pulmonary hypertension is an increase in blood pressure in the pulmonary arteries, veins, and capillaries that supply the lungs. Once again, the symptoms overlap with the symptoms of other heart problems and with the symptoms of COPD, so keep your doctor abreast of all your breathing problems.

Your doctor might want you to have an ECG (echocardiogram) or stress test to help diagnose a heart problem. Keep your heart healthy through diet, adherence to proper medications, medically approved exercise, and using your O2 when and if it is ordered by your doctor. Hey, I warned you that managing your COPD is a full-time job!

High or Low Red Blood Cell Counts
Red blood cells carry O2 to our muscles and organs. Chronic O2 deprivation can cause an increase in our red blood cell count (called polycythemia or "thick blood"). It sure is a good reason to use your

O2 if it is prescribed! Smoking can also cause an increase in red blood count. (If you are still a smoker, you can insert your own lecture here; just be sure to make it severe!) Ironically, COPD can also cause low red blood cell counts (anemia). This may be due to the inflammatory aspect of COPD. Red blood cells need iron, so be sure you get blood tests to determine the status of your blood and iron. Don't take iron supplements without talking to your doctor. Too much iron can cause serious problems, too!

GERD (gastro esophageal reflux disease) or Acid Reflux
I don't know if we are more prone to acid reflux (or GERD/gastro esophageal reflux disease) than other people, but it sure is common among COPDers! Burning discomfort, chest discomfort, difficulty swallowing, and waking up at night having regurgitated (often up to one's mouth) are all symptoms of acid reflux. Often overlooked is that it can also cause a chronic cough! Reflux is especially dangerous for us because of the chance of inhaling small foreign particles of reflux (or even fumes) into our lungs. It is believed that COPD patients with acid reflux have more exacerbations than those who do not have it. If you have a reflux problem, talk to your doctor about treatment.

Thrush
Thrush is a yeast infection, usually of the mouth. The yeast *(Candida albicans)* is normally found in various parts of the body but is kept in check. Rinsing and gargling each time you use your inhaler or nebulizer containing a steroid (technically, a corticosteroid) goes a long way in preventing thrush. The use of antibiotics can also lead to thrush. The combination of both antibiotics and corticosteroid medications, often used by those of us with COPD, can especially upset the natural balance of microorganisms in our body—a balance that would ordinarily prevent the yeast from getting out of hand. Yes, we've messed with Mother Nature. It often feels like a sore mouth or throat and has the appearance of little white patches. Report any symptoms to your doctor (whether or not you see white patches), who can treat it with medications, often lozenges, oral rinses, or pills. You may be able to prevent thrush by eating yogurt that contains live cultures of acidophilus (don't freeze or cook the yogurt). Just be sure it says "live" on the container. You can also buy the acidophilus in capsules or lozenges (check to see if they require refrigeration after the bottle

is opened). Consider making a yogurt smoothie using fresh or frozen berries, yogurt, and a bit of water to thin it out.

Cataracts

Cataracts are the clouding of the eye's lens that leads to poor vision. COPD does not cause cataracts, but continued use of oral corticosteroid medications can. Inhaled corticosteroids are probably not a problem. If you think you may be developing cataracts, buying a larger screen TV and relying on your car horn more often is not the preferred way with which to deal with this impairment! Removal of cataracts is now a simple procedure, even for those of us with advanced COPD.

Sleep Apnea

A large number of people with COPD also have sleep apnea; I don't know why. Sleep apnea means that you stop breathing when sleeping. That's serious. There are two types, and the type more common for us with COPD is obstructive sleep apnea, in which the soft tissue at the rear of the throat collapses during sleep and breathing stops, sometimes hundreds of times a night. Untreated sleep apnea is very serious as it can lead to fatigue, sleepiness during the day, memory problems, high blood pressure, and cardiovascular problems. The symptoms of sleep apnea are very loud snoring, non refreshing sleep, and excessive daytime sleepiness—a tendency to nod off inadvertently when sitting quietly. Sleepiness while reading this book is not a symptom. Sleep apnea can be treated, once properly diagnosed, with airway pressure machines, called CPAP machines, that keep your airway passages open while you sleep.

Diabetes

I know quite a few people with COPD and diabetes. I don't know if diabetes is due to the lifestyles commonly adopted by people with COPD or if it is something else, but there are quite a few of us with both! The use of oral steroids (corticosteroids) sometimes leads to or contributes to diabetes and some of us with COPD end up on oral doses of corticosteroids. Most people know that diabetes is a problem with the body's regulation of sugar. If untreated it can cause very serious damage, including cardiac problems, loss of limbs, blindness… have I scared you enough? Report any of the following symptoms:

excessive thirst, frequent urination, extreme hunger, unusual weight loss, irritability, or blurred vision.

Incontinence

People with COPD sometimes ask if it causes incontinence. The answer is that there are many causes to incontinence, so it needs to be checked out by your doctor. But, yes, if your O2 saturation temporarily goes too low, your body needs to protect vital organs from the lack of O2. In its effort to protect some organs, like your brain, it gives them priority by allocating more blood and O2 to them at the expense of others, such as your bladder or muscles involved in the bladder or bowels. With less O2, they just don't work as well. It is very discouraging to have this problem. Incontinence products are available for both men and women for both bladder and bowel control problems.

Memory Problems

Memory problems are common complaints of people with COPD. Usually, the complaints concern the inability to hold things long enough in short-term memory. It is important to know that we're all getting older, too, and it is hard to tease the two possible co-conspirators apart! It is more common for the memory loss to be just annoying, the type of thing you'd joke about. At other times it can be severe enough to be quite upsetting. So, do memory problems come along with COPD? Well, yes and no. Research says COPD "might" affect our memory and cognition. Some people with COPD develop memory problems, but some do not. Those who are affected can usually use a few common tricks, such as writing things down, check lists, maintaining strict organization, etc., to compensate. The older you get and more advanced your COPD becomes, the greater the chance you will have some problems. Also, any major illnesses, depression, lack of simulation, and medications can affect memory, so you are not going to be able to diagnose or adequately address memory problems by reading a self-help book, including this one. If you are having memory problems, the first thing you need to do is talk to your doctor about it.

Depression and Anxiety

Yes, depression and anxiety disorders (including panic disorders) are serious secondary illnesses and very common with people with COPD. For example, between 25% and 50% of people with COPD report being depressed. You will find chapters devoted to these illnesses ahead.

Flatulence

Don't think for a minute you can blame your excessive farting on COPD! It has nothing to do with it! Use the excuse if you must with your friends and family, but the rest of us COPDers know better! Okay, I'll give you this: When we are SOB, many of us swallow more air than usual, so if you want to use COPD as an excuse for belching, you can get away with it. However, this does not give you permission to engage in preadolescent belching contests!

Chapter 18

GETTING OUT, MOBILITY, AND TRAVELING

Travel and change of place impart new vigor to the mind.
~ Seneca

Keeping physically active is very important. Looking for the remote control is not considered a planned physical exercise program. Physical activity is not only good for your body, it is also good for your mind. It is easy and even tempting to withdraw from activity when it seems to take more and more effort to get out and about. Also, some of us get so tired of having to cancel our plans because we are having bad breathing days that we find ourselves making fewer commitments. Friends and family occasionally give up inviting or encouraging us to socialize with them, sometimes out of frustration and sometimes because they simply don't want to burden us. Add all of these up, and include dealing with extremes in weather, and it results in many reasons to just stay at home. The problem is that this retreat from activity outside our homes isn't good for us. We easily begin to spiral downward—lack of activity leads to us to become out of shape, which makes our breathing more difficult, which in turn leads to less activity, which leads to—well, you see, a vicious downward spiral! We have to constantly fight against that happening to us. Some of us win the battle and stay remarkably active, and it is just part of our lifestyle, whereas others of us have to push ourselves more.

There are very few things that could be more beneficial to us than participating in respiratory rehab therapy. If you haven't already done so, ask your doctor about getting into a rehab program. Additionally, check your area for local support groups where you can not only socialize with others and get peer support, but also learn more about management of your disease and, equally important, share your tips with others. Ask your doctor, local pulmonary rehabilitation center, or local hospital if there is a support group in your area. If there aren't any, consider starting one.

Accommodations for Those of Us with Disabilities

Be aware that the Americans with Disabilities Act (ADA) literally opens doors for us. Those of us with "significant" breathing impairments cannot be discriminated against in employment (covered earlier), state and local governments and services, public accommodations, transportation, and telecommunications. Much of what follows concerning our mobility and opportunities to travel has been influenced, if not mandated, by the ADA.

Participation in Your Community and Public Accommodations

The ADA requires businesses to provide reasonable accommodation to people with disabilities and prohibits exclusion of people with handicaps from activities such as getting medical services, shopping, enjoying a movie, dining out, joining a health club, or using any service provider in the community. State and local governments must provide an equal opportunity for those of us who have a disability due to our COPD to benefit from all of their programs, services, and activities offered. Specifically, you should be accommodated when it comes to voting, education, health care, government programs, recreation programs, social services, and transportation. The important catchword for all accommodation measures is that they should be "reasonable." If it is too costly or difficult to provide accommodation, no one is required to accommodate those of us with a disability.

> ADA Information Line
> (800) 514-0301 (voice)
> (800) 514-0383 (TTY)
> www.ada.gov

Local Public Transportation

Some states and communities do better in meeting the needs of transportation for people with disabilities than others. However, don't take anything for granted. Call your local department of transportation to find out what is available to you. These agencies often don't go around advertising what is available, so you might need to take the initiative to find out what is available.

Driving and Parking

When you feel the need, you can get either disability license plates through your department of motor vehicles or a handicap tag you can hang from your rearview mirror from your local municipality. Either will require documentation from your doctor. Even if you do not have a car, it is useful to have a handicapped tag so whoever is driving you can park in a handicapped spot as long as you are with them. Because of the parking advantages, you might find that you are invited out more often. However, don't assume that handicapped parking means convenient parking. It is sometimes necessary to "scope out" places before making plans to go there. You can't believe what people tell you on the phone when they say, "Sure, parking is right outside the door."

The ADA requires that gas stations pump gas for us at our request *if* more than one station assistant is present. If this is the case, the station can only charge us the cost of the gas that is self-serve. The problem is, few gas station workers seem to know this law, and when you wave them over, they wave back as they try to figure out who you are.

States seem to handle the renewal of driver's licenses for people on portable O2 differently. Anecdotal stories report that it is absolutely no issue in some states, while other states require doctor's reports that vary in length and require details and determinations such as how far from home the person on O2 is allowed to drive.

Local Activities

Support Groups

Many locales have support groups for people with asthma and COPD. Contact your local American Lung Association to find out if there are any near you.

Religious Groups

Religion and attending religious services is an important part of many people's lives. There are often groups and meetings within your religious organization that provide opportunities to socialize.

Shopping

Malls, especially during the weekday when they are less crowded, provide great climate control and often have adequate seating. Large grocery stores can also be great places to walk, not only because they, too, are climate controlled, but also because they have carts. Many of us can walk much further with a cart than we can without one. A rule of thumb for COPDers is that you should try to topple at least one display a week as part of your exercise routine.

Casinos

How many activities can you do while sitting, where no one cares how you are dressed, that is distracting to the eyes and ears, doesn't require thinking, does not involve consuming food, offends no one when you get up and leave out of frustration, and provides all of this with valet service?

Social Centers

Many locales have social centers for older people, and even if you aren't an older person, you might be able to get in. They are managed by local government agencies or community centers. They serve as a great gathering place for people with limited mobility and those who need opportunities for social interactions. The centers often have courses or provide training in arts, crafts, and hobbies. Just be careful to choose activities that don't involve odors.

Adult Classes

Consider taking an adult class or two. They are often available through the community centers mentioned above and also available at local colleges, libraries, etc. Keeping the mind active is very important. Learn something new.

Movies

Hey, you are probably able to go during the day when it is less crowded, quieter, and cheaper!

Sporting Events and Concerts

You might not do as much cheering as you used to, and you certainly aren't going to climb too high into the bleachers, but your COPD doesn't have to stop you from watching your favorite sports. When you purchase tickets, ask for the seats for people with handicaps and find out their location. Often, they are choice seats. Get out and support your local teams!

Swimming

Swimming is a fantastic, low-impact exercise that can include water aerobics. Just be sure you can tolerate the chlorine. Don't take you O2 equipment in the water or create a hazard with your tubing.

Bowling

You just might be able to do this, and it uses a lot of different muscle groups!

Yoga or Tai Chi

There are many types of such practices to choose from that are good for both the mind and the body. They should be very seriously considered, and they might open new doors for you.

Strip Clubs

I'm just checking to see if you are paying attention! Well, actually, now that I'm thinking about it...

Museums

With good planning, you can avoid the crowds. Museums usually have good climate control, adequate seating, and abundant inspiration.

Gardening and Gardening Clubs

Gardening is a popular activity; just be careful of inhaling fumes, dust, and other things involved in gardening.

Volunteering

Yes, you might not be able to work, but you might be able to handle a couple of hours a week doing something meaningful. Avoid volunteering where sick people congregate!

Long-Distance Travel
Airline Travel
If you use supplemental O2, read be sure to read the chapter on oxygen. If you are not on O2, double check with your doctor to be sure you can safely travel on a plane. The cabin, although pressurized, is not pressurized to sea level, and you might need supplemental O2 during the flight.

Rail Travel
People rave about their rail trips, although not many people take them. Rail lines are required to have handicapped facilities, and some trains have rooms with sleeping accommodations, including private toilets and showers. Not all train stops are handicapped accessible. Call Amtrak, (800) USA-RAIL, or visit www.amtrak.com for more information.

Commercial Bus Travel
This can be a good option if the distance isn't too long.

RV Travel
What a way to travel, especially if you can afford a motorized Class A vehicle! A Class A motorized vehicle has the living area within the same area as the driver and passenger seats. There are companies that rent a variety of RVs for vacation travel.

Cruise Ship Travel
Cruise ships can be a wonderful way to spend a vacation as long as you occasionally leave your seat at the buffet. It is always embarrassing when they have to ask you to take your chair back to the table. Although there are special cruises for people with COPD, traditional cruise ships should not be ruled out; larger ones have a doctor and medical facilities on board. Whether or not the ADA covers cruise ships that fly foreign flags (most ships) remains unclear in spite of numerous split-decision court cases. Newer ships tend to be designed to be more accommodating than older ships.

Travel Insurance
Check your medical insurance to determine what coverage you have (if any) once you leave the United States. Medicare's coverage is

extremely limited. If you leave the United States, you should consider travel insurance, but search high and low for one that doesn't exclude prior existing conditions. It might be a very difficult search, and you may need a travel agent for a recommendation, but insurance coverage that does not exclude preexisting conditions *Is* out there!

Find Time to Get Out

Free yourself up as much as possible from some of the mundane tasks that need to be completed in order to make the time and have the energy needed to get out and enjoy life! Sometimes just keeping up with necessary household chores is about all some of us can handle. Any shortcuts we can learn to make those tasks easier are helpful.

Chapter 19

TIPS FOR MAKING PHYSICAL ACTIVITIES EASIER

I'm not going to vacuum until Sears makes one you can ride on.
~Roseanne Barr

As COPD progresses, our ability to take care of ourselves and our homes becomes more challenging. We need ways to make the most of what physical ability we still have. Trying to conserve your energy will lead you to create many shortcuts to make your life easier. In many cases you may not have to recreate the wheel.

Besides just keeping up with necessary chores, being able to take care of ourselves is very important to us emotionally as well; we must, therefore, fight to remain functioning as independently as possible (without becoming stubborn). It takes very little for things to start becoming overwhelming. Keeping up with your personal needs and the household chores will help you feel in control. It is hard to feel "up" when you are stuck in the middle of an indoor slum, or feel strong when things around you are out of control.

We must also face the reality that there might be a time when we are unable to take care of ourselves or our homes without assistance from others. When and if this happens to you, don't blame yourself; remember, it is the disease imposing this upon you, and it is not your fault. On the bright side, if there is one, getting to this point means you've outlived many others who have not made it this far. There are three basic rules for making the most of what we have:

1. **Always Trade Up**
   Being active is very important, but you don't want to squander your limited supply of energy or use it all up on mundane chores. Economize as much as you can when attending to the "must do's" so that you still have energy left for enjoyable activities.

   Eventually, for some of us trying to perform our necessary activities, even using our tips and shortcuts will be too taxing on us. Many states have programs to provide assistance with basic chores, such as assistance in bathing, light housekeeping, and shopping. Not all states are the same or equal when it comes to services available through Medicare. Although it is a federal program, it is administered by individual states, and they differ when it comes to what is covered. There are often state and local resources available, so check them out. They sometimes require that you be sixty-two or sixty-five, but sometimes it is based upon age *or* disability.

2. **Timing is Everything!**
   For many of us, *when* we choose to do our chores, exercise, or do physical tasks is important; you'll probably have to pick your best part of the day.

3. **Pace It and Space It!**
   Pace yourself. This, for us, always means slowing down. Early on in our disease, it is common for many, if not most of us, to have picked up the bad habit of sprinting. Learn to move and walk more slowly and take more breaks along the way. Stop and take a rest before, not after, you become out of breath. Remind yourself you are now a tortoise and not a hare.

   Scheduling chores allows you to space them out better. Wait for a decent- enough day during the week to complete the one or two tasks scheduled for that week. Larger tasks, like reorganizing a closet or cleaning the garage, can be scheduled for a particular month. Just give yourself a break; most things can wait if you stop and think about it. Avoid overwhelming projects such as "clean the whole house." Just spread the projects out and then pace yourself within each task.

Tips for Common Routines
  Sleeping and Bedroom Set-up
  1. **Get a Good Mattress**
     A good night of sleep is very important. A good night's sleep will make everything easier!

  2. **Choose the Right Bed**
     Consider an adjustable bed. Sleeping with your head raised often helps some of us breathe. It is often also recommended

for individuals with acid reflux disease. Check to see if your condition medically qualifies you for an adjustable hospital bed through your insurance company.

3. **Nightstands**
   Arrange all the things you will need during the night and upon first waking next to your bed. Throw out that annoying little nightstand I know you have and get something larger!

4. **Urinating at Night**
   First of all, be sure to get out of bed, walk to the bathroom, and then pee in the correct order. Better, consider using a portable urinal. Stumbling around at night can be hazardous, and many accidents occur tripping on entangled bedding or O2 hoses while getting out of bed. Also, tell your doctor if you are urinating frequently.

5. **Making Your Bed**
   You'd be surprised how much of the bed you can make while lying in it, so do as much as you can while still in it. Avoid heavy blankets and coverings. Think of it as airing out the bed during the day by not making it!

Bathing, Shaving, and Oral Care

1. **Make Your Bathroom Handicapped-Friendly!**
   Do you need your toilet raised? If so, there are products that fit right over your existing toilet to raise it up to make it more comfortable for some people. Are there hand rails where you need them? Don't wait until you need them to have them installed. Always look ahead. Check the Internet under "handicapped bathing" or "disability equipment," and you'll find many great ideas!

2. **Reevaluate and Economize Your Bathing Routine!**
   Take a serious look at your current routine to see if it can be modified. We sometimes stick to old routines simply out of habit; hey, that's why they are called routines! There is no rule that says that you have to get dressed right after bathing or even get dressed in the bathroom. Women might want to throw (okay, gently place) all their cosmetics in an attractive

wooden box next to their most comfortable and well-lit sitting area so that they can comfortably slap on (okay, apply) all that beauty crap (okay, products) in relative comfort.

3. **Get Rid of the Humidity!**
   Bathing or showering is one of the more difficult things for many of us. Not only is it a lot of physical work, but the heat and humidity can do us in. My rule is that if I can do nothing else for the rest of the day, bathing is my number one priority, and I'll take as long as needed to accomplish it. As humidity is often a problem, you may need to experiment a bit by manipulating the following things:

   - Open a window if you have one.

   - Keep the door to the bathroom ajar, if not totally open.

   - Use a small fan to create a current (consider a battery-operated fan).

   - Create an air current within the shower area by opening the curtain a crack—just be careful where you point the handheld showerhead.

   - Keep the temperature of the water lower if you have a serious fog problem.

4. **Dress and Undress in Stages!**
   Take your time. Yes, you can dress and undress in stages. If sitting on your commode is not comfortable, consider a comfortable chair in the bathroom if you have the space. Remember to rest after each step.

5. **Rub-a-Dub-Dub, Tips for the Tub!**
   - Make believe you are getting paid by the hour and don't like your employer—stretch it out a bit, or a lot!

   - If you use O2, simply throw the tubing over the shower rod. Ask your doctor what setting you can use for strenuous activities of short duration, such as bathing.

   - If you don't have a shower chair, get one!

- Use a handheld showerhead and bathe from the top down. Women find that they can wash their hair in the shower with their head tilted back—far better, for many, than hanging their head over a sink. Many women with COPD discover the benefits of short hair.

- Keep all your soaps and bathing supplies within reach, and install a shelf if you have to. Try non scented products if you are sensitive to odors.

- Open the curtain or door periodically to help the steam escape. Don't wait for it to be overwhelming.

- Consider sponges or brushes on sticks, or one of those battery-operated brushes you see advertised on TV that twirl around and eat up batteries.

6. **Dry Yourself Off!**
Be sure to use a bathmat so you don't slip getting out of the shower. Some days, bathing can be quite an accomplishment (but your friends and family will be happy that you did). Consider buying a nice terrycloth robe (but not a heavy one). Instead of toweling off, you can wrap it around you and slowly pat yourself dry. Be sure to give your robe a chance to thoroughly dry between showers.

7. **Comb Your Hair and Brush Your Teeth!**
There is no rule that says you have to do these at the same time you are completing your showering or bathing routine. Consider brushing your teeth before your shower when it is less humid.

- Electric or battery toothbrushes are very handy.

- Either change your toothbrush regularly or consider ways to disinfect your brush, especially after an illness. UV (ultraviolet) sanitizers for use with manual and electric brushes are now available at a reasonable price.

- Consider a water floss machine.

- A chair in front of the sink with a mirror propped behind the faucet allows you to sit while brushing or shaving.

- O2 users are warned not to use ANY electrical appliance while using O2, including electric shavers and hair dryers.

Dressing
Dress Comfortably!
Here are a few tips.

- Avoid tight fitting clothing, especially around your waist.

- Drawstrings make dressing easier.

- Suspenders are better than belts.

- Slip-ons or Velcro fastened shoes help you avoid bending over, a motion that seems to get us especially SOB.

- Avoid clothing that goes on over the head.

- Camisoles and sports bras are more comfortable than regular bras. Men who look like they need a bra should not take their shirts off in public!

- Diabetic socks are preferable for both men and women.

- Putting your underwear inside your pants before putting them on can save you an extra step. Just be sure the underwear is on the *inside*!

- Rearranging where you store your clothing can help minimize bending.

Shopping and Schlepping
1. Don't Collapse!
Use a collapsible shopping cart instead. The ones with swivel front wheels, sometimes a bit hard to find, are much more versatile. They can be stored in the trunk of your car and used to transport groceries or other items. If you load it with groceries, you can pull it right up to your refrigerator.

2. Keep Cool!
When grocery shopping, pack all your frozen or refrigerated food in the same bag so that you can get them stored first and then worry about the other things later.

3. **Keep on Rollin'!**

    For individuals more challenged by other ailments or who
    have more advanced COPD, a rollator might be your solution.
    A rollator is a foldable walker on wheels but is usually much
    sturdier and has hand brakes not unlike a bicycle. Most have
    a small basket for storage, and they are available with a seat
    that appears when you unfold it. Some even come with cup
    holders—handy for begging on the street to help pay for your
    expensive meds.

4. **Climb Your Way Up!**

    Stairs can be a huge challenge, especially when carrying some-
    thing. Exhale, place the object you are carrying up a couple of
    stairs, rest, walk up a few stairs, rest again, and repeat the pro-
    cess. You can curse the disease on each third step if you like.

5. **Move it!**

    I've read about recommendations to use carts with multiple
    shelves for moving things around when doing housework,
    and if you are organized and think things through, it can be a
    great advantage.

6. **You Send Me!**

    Consider using the Internet for shopping. Larger orders of
    things such as drug store items often have free shipping.
    Consider pharmacy by mail; you can sometimes even save
    money, because many insurance companies will give you a
    significant discount if you order a three-month supply from
    their partner companies.

Cleaning

1. **Use Your Influence!**

    Identify all close friends and family members who are able
    to do your cleaning. Take each one aside individually and tell
    them that they are your sole heir, but that you will change the
    will if they tell anyone. Your house will be kept spotless.

2. **Help!**

    If you can afford it, hire help to clean your home if the above
    suggestion doesn't work.

3. **Avoid All Fumes!**

Remember that there is no natural law that says all dangerous fumes must have an odor. Chemicals with mild or no odor can also be damaging or irritating to your lungs.

4. **Danger!**

People using O2 should not use aerosol products. Actually, none of us should!

5. **Good on Salads, Too!**

Plain white vinegar is fine for most cleaning projects. Vinegar is championed as an effective disinfectant that also deodorizes, cuts grease and soap scum, inhibits molds and dissolves minerals. Be aware that it might dissolve grout and do not use it on marble as it will start to dissolve it. Many people use it in a spray bottle. If used full strength, it is supposed to kill 99% of bacteria; however, the fumes can be too strong. You can also dilute the vinegar by an equal amount of water.

6. **Clean Au Naturale!**

Get your mind out of the gutter! I'm not talking about cleaning naked, I'm talking about using baking soda, a natural substance that absorbs orders and is a good mild abrasive! A few drops of water or vinegar added to the baking soda makes a nice paste for cleaning tubs, sinks, counters, etc.

7. **What a Lemon!**

I've read recommendations to avoid lemon-scented soaps or cleaning products. I'm not sure why. Perhaps it has to do with the use of oils in the products.

Vacuuming

1. **Avoid Dust!**

Dust is worse when floating through the air than it is safely resting on the floor. If you see your footprints as you walk indoors, however, it might be time to vacuum. Consider a using a mask or relative.

2. Get a Robot!
The motorized self-directed robot vacuums (Rumba or other brands, if there are any) actually have good reputations for doing a decent job!

3. Hit and Run!
If you cajole someone into vacuuming, leave the room while they are at work. Do not point out spots they missed from a distance, or do so only when disguising your voice.

4. Get an Old Bag to Help You Vacuum!
Forget the "bagless" vacuums; they are a mess to empty, and that's the last stuff you need to inhale. Stick with the older disposable-bag models.

5. Call on the Carpet!
If I had my druthers, I'd get rid of all carpeting and only have hardwood or tile floors; they are much easier to keep clean.

Dusting
1. Perform Magic with a Wand!
Use one of those static magic-wand disposable dusters. They work. Don't shake it out to clean it, just replace it.

2. Need a Reminder?
If you don't get around to dusting, use dusty surfaces to leave reminder notes.

Laundry
1. Have a Seat!
Sitting on a short stool will help you reach into your machines if they are the annoying front-loading type.

2. Get a Grasp!
The mechanical reacher-grabber-picker-upper-pincher on a stick is invaluable for many things and especially useful for moving laundry around.

3. **Get Outta Here!**
   Call around to all of your local Laundromats to find out if any of them offer pickup and delivery.

4. **Look for Alternatives!**
   You won't have to worry about laundry as often if you join a nudist colony. In addition, I'm sure your O2 supply company will be delighted to make daily deliveries if necessary.

Painting

Stay away from all types of chemicals! Get someone else to do your painting and insist they only use paint that is labeled "zero VOC paint (or primer)." VOC stands for "volatile organic compounds," the vapors that are release into the air as it dries.

Cooking

If you use portable O2, you must read the chapter on oxygen. These tips are not written with the O2 user in mind, even though some of the tips can be very useful.

1. **Get Organized!**
   Organize your kitchen for convenience and not esthetics.

2. **Scale Down!**
   You might find that small countertop convection ovens/toasters are extremely convenient as well as efficient. They are also easier to clean than most ovens.

3. **Move It!**
   If you have a small kitchen, consider getting an armless office chair. You can adjust the height for your comfort and be seated while you prep food, load the dishwasher, etc. Just be careful that it does not wreck your floors. Be extremely careful not to let it slip out from under you when you bend over or are about to sit.

4. **Unload Your Burden.**
   Unload the dishwasher in stages. Stack the dishes on the countertop above your dishwasher and, once they are all arranged, put them where they are typically stored.

5. **Take Small Bites!**

   Making a meal from start to finish might be biting off more than you can chew. Prep your evening meal in the afternoon, and then have everything in place for cooking later.

6. **Stuff It!**

   As long as you are cooking, make enough to freeze for quick meals. If you have a rare good breathing day, consider preparing foods to stuff in your freezer for another day.

7. **Start Giving Orders!**

   If shopping for food is a problem, you can order your groceries online in some areas of the country. You can shop online, browse the aisles, and have items delivered at your convenience. Internet access is required, and all you have to do is look up the Web sites for the larger chain grocery stores in your area to see if delivery service is available. There are also companies that will ship even fresh food via one of the national delivery services.

Help with Cooking

The last thing someone with COPD needs is a fire (and smoke), even a small one—or any other kind of accident in the kitchen, for that matter! Here are some tips that just might prevent an accident:

- Your clothing should not be loose or flowing because it increases the likelihood that it could catch fire. Bare arms are best.

- Don't store cooking oils or alcohol near the stove or any open flame.

- Don't spray cooking oils into a pan when there is a flame under or near it, and certainly don't flambé anything!

- Keep potholders away from the flame and do not use kitchen towels for potholders.

- Do not stick your head over anything on the stove.

- Do not set the flame so high that it flows over and up the side of the pan.

- Maintain a stiff posture away from the stove while cooking.

- Do not leave potholders on the lids while they are on the stove.

- Kitchen towels should be returned to their racks, a distance from the stove.

- Don't yak it up on the phone or watch TV while you are cooking at the stove.

- Keep at least one ABC fire extinguisher readily available. Use an extra dose of common sense when it comes to deciding whether to even try to put out a fire. Remember that your lungs are compromised!

For Those Who Can't Cook
For those who do not cook or are unable to cook, frozen meals have come a long way and are worth retesting (pay attention to the sodium content, though). Also check out a local Meals on Wheels program to see if you are eligible. You may even consider the meals offered through weight loss programs that advertise on TV and which are delivered to your door. You can always add a bit to them, but you will be getting basic, well-balanced nutrition. In addition, I've heard of many people praising a company called Schwans, which delivers quality frozen foods (www.schwans.com or 1-888-SCHWANS) in many areas. There is also another company, www.netgrocer.com, that ships groceries right to your door via a major carrier like UPS or FedEx! And, yes, they now can even send frozen foods!

As we struggle to get things done and use as many shortcuts and tips as possible, there are moments when we sit back and wonder how the heck we got into this situation and what is happening to us. Having COPD is not just about making physical accommodations to our growing limitations, it is also about adjusting emotionally to this difficult journey.

Chapter 20

WHAT HAPPENED TO ME AND WHO AM I NOW?

If you don't like something, change it; if you can't change it, change the way you think about it.
~Mary Engelbreit

Why Me?

Let's start off with a big question: Why did you get COPD and not someone else? No, I don't mean the smoking issue if you were a smoker. When you smoked, you were just hedging your bets that you could be one of those many people (about 80%) who get away with smoking and do not get COPD. That'll teach you to gamble! Actually, probably unknown to you was that your genes put you at higher risk than other smokers who didn't get COPD. But why did you end up with those lousy genes? Why did *you*, out of many others, end up with an incurable, nasty disease? I bet you believe one of the following:

1. **Lesson to learn**: You believe that your illness was designed by a higher power and that there are lessons for you to learn from this experience.

2. **Punishment**: Your disease was doled out to you as a punishment for some indiscretion in this or a past life.

3. **Luck of the Draw**: It was just the result of a lousy, random, impersonal draw of the cards.

What you believe has everything to do with how you'll cope with this disease. Your philosophy will be the foundation upon which you will build coping skills. Sure, you may bounce around in your belief, but there is probably one of the above that most accurately describes you. Here's how your belief will affect you:

Lessons to Learn (Fate)

Many of us believe that there is a purpose or plan for us behind our suffering, and our "challenge" or "fate" is the creation of a higher power. The reason for this plan may or may not also be known to us—in other words, "for everything there is a reason." Some of us will search for the meaning of why we are being tested in this manner, while others of us believe that it is beyond our ability to understand the reason. With this philosophy or belief system comes a level of acceptance that can help us to cope, because we do not see ourselves as victims. If you believe that you have COPD for a reason, you will probably benefit in the following ways by having:

- a lack of guilt because your illness was "meant to be";

- an acceptance of your illness;

- a guiding belief or philosophy to help you through the many rough times;

- moments of inspiration or insight;

- motivation to move ahead;

- faith that it is possible for you to deal with or overcome obstacles;

- greater opportunities to experience a sense of mastery when you overcome obstacles;

- less intense or fewer feelings of anger or feeling victimized.

Punishment

Some of us simply feel guilty over everything! For us, having COPD not only feels like a punishment, we believe deep down that it is a punishment—because that's how it feels. We are pissed and angry—not just once in a while but most of the time! This self-blame racket is usually a lifelong trait (unless you put an end to it), even though you might protest to the contrary and even lash out in denial on occasion. When self-blame is a mind-set, you are predisposed to blame yourself for your COPD as soon as you got the diagnosis. When guilt or blame takes root in such fertile ground, it is time to do some weeding! If you can accept that your COPD might be your big chance to change how you feel about yourself, and therefore your value and importance in this world, then you have found a purpose. In doing so, you are not letting COPD make a victim of you. The choice is yours. Yes, you do have a choice.

Luck of the Draw

There are a large number of us who are not going to hold higher powers responsible for our COPD. No, there are no spiritual quests, opportunities to transcend mortal suffering, or any heavenly design involved in singling us out. We are not personally responsible for our COPD and believe it means nothing more than having been dealt a crappy hand of cards or having randomly received some incorrigible genes. Having been dealt a crappy hand doesn't mean that the next card won't be better (or worse), but for the most part, the ante has already been paid. You therefore might as well stay in the game and play your hand the best you can and make the best of it. Be aware that when you give up the focus on either winning or losing, you can better enjoy the game and the company of other players.

As you are trying to figure out or justify why you have COPD, you are often doing so while your life is dramatically changing. It is not unlike trying to tie your shoes while you are walking. One of the biggest changes that occurs in our life, and which for us is usually related to our illness, is saying goodbye to our jobs, careers, and coworkers, and being forced to accept a new stage of life and adjust to a new lifestyle—a new lifestyle we will call "retirement."

The New You: Adjusting to Retirement

If you are still working, you are probably already worried about how much longer you are going to be able to work. If you have retired, not because of your age but because of your disability, it is a mixed blessing. If you were already retired when you were first hit with COPD, it probably has changed your expectations of the rest of your retirement years, perhaps even robbed you of some of the activities you had planned. Feeling robbed of the "golden years" is a tremendous loss. I want to point out that if you feel robbed, you are feeling victimized. See how your belief about why you got COPD is important? Nevertheless, we can all feel cheated, and the onset of feelings of loss, grief, and even depression often surprises people.

Retirement, whether it is voluntary or due to disability, is a lot more than just giving up work. Retirement changes our role in life and how we not only see ourselves but also how others see us. Somehow or another, we are no longer associated with what we used to do for a living. In our society, "What do you do for a living?" is one of the first questions asked. It defines who we are. Our identity is changing on us! Help! Some changes that take place upon retirement are predictable, and others catch some of us by surprise. We discover new things about ourselves, both pleasant and unpleasant.

One of the biggest changes is that when we worked, we had routines, expectations, and demands placed upon us. We were very much controlled from the outside. Our lives were structured. We had to be at work at a set time, and we had to go to bed around a specific time to get enough sleep. Our weekends were often structure to meet the demands upon us, and the only real rest from structure was those vacations that ended just as we were beginning to really feel relaxed. Not only were we structured, our jobs came with expectations: output was measured and evaluated, and we were rewarded or punished accordingly. Further, we often spent more time with work projects and co-workers than we did with our own families!

Our brain needs to adapt to the lack of stimulation—both good and bad stimulation—that often accompanies retirement. We now may have to actually go out of our way at times to find or create structure! Ugh! We miss problems to solve, challenges to face, new things to learn, social interactions, and, most important, receiving rewards and acknowledgements. Who would have thought we'd miss these things when all we really wanted was a break from it all, to rest? Who would have ever expected that work and structure were addictive and that our minds would actually develop a need for them?

Yes, it is time for some tips for adjusting to this new way of life.

Tips for Retirement

Most "retirement tips" out there have to do with financial planning. You'll find nothing here about financial planning. I failed financial planning. However, I do have some pointers on how to add value to your retirement that have little to do with money.

The first thing you need to do upon retirement (forced upon you due to COPD or otherwise) is to sit back and rest for a bit. When the seat on your lawn chair starts to sag so low you need assistance getting out of it, or you follow people around talking to them despite their best efforts to avoid you, it is time to take action. Outside of sex during the middle of the day, here are some other things you can do:

Maintain Some Structure

Give yourself some daily structure—yes, structure for the sake of structure. Remember that your brain has become addicted to structure. You don't have to be a taskmaster. Sure, you can change your plans in midstream if you want, but give yourself something to change.

Stay Active

Remaining active, both physically and mentally, is imperative. It is one of the few things you can do for both your mental and physical health, now more than ever. Seriously consider a physical exercise routine—yes, routine! Check with your doctor about your exercise routine and get his or her approval before starting.

Stay Social

We may not think social interactions mean much to us, but they are important. If you stop and count up the average number of interactions you had with others on the job, even if it is a brief nod or "hello," you might be astounded. Your mate, if you have one, usually cannot compensate (or shouldn't have to compensate) for the lack of social interaction. Go out and make new friends. If you can't physically get out, get on the Internet.

Keep Learning

Do not retire your brain; you are going to need it as much in the future as ever—maybe more! Learn new things and keep learning. Doing crossword puzzles every day is great and challenging, but not quite varied enough to exercise all of your brain. The brain needs a variety of activities as well as challenges that stretch it and work it like all the muscles in your body.

Be Useful

We can forget how important being useful is. I don't mean just being useful around the house and knocking off a couple of house maintenance projects, I'm talking about doing something to add to or enrich the lives of others!

Enjoy Hobbies

I put hobbies at the bottom of the list if for no other reason than they are usually put at the top of the list of "what to do" when one retires! Hobbies can be part of any of the above list of things, such as learning something new, or can stand alone. Hobbies often allow you to complete something—a good feeling we sometimes miss. If looking for a hobby or craft, stay away from those that entail smelling fumes, dust, etc., that might irritate your lungs.

Yes, retirement due to COPD can be a blessing for some, a curse for others, or even a mixed blessing. Be mindful not to get engulfed by your own needs. Having COPD is not just about us; it is about how our illness affects our families, especially our mates.

Watching them struggle coming to terms with your illness and the impact it might have on both of you can be stressful, frightening, and painful. Further, they are the ones who are "supposed" to "be there" for you during your time of need, but frankly, some spouses will "be there" and some won't. The right thing to do is to understand what they might be going through, how your illness might affect your relationship, and what, if anything, you can do to minimize the damage that COPD creates.

Chapter 21

SPOUSES AND PARTNERS OF PEOPLE WITH COPD

The goal in marriage is not to think alike, but to think together.
~*Robert C. Dodds*

Like it or not, your partner is going to have to deal one way or another with your COPD. Your illness might affect his or her life almost as much as it does yours, only in different ways. Your partner can be your ally, friend, caretaker, and support, or he or she can abandon you emotionally, physically, or both. Your partner's reaction has everything to do with your history together, your choice of partner, or how "stewed" you were when you proposed or accepted the proposal. Regardless of your choice of partner, you probably have come to realize by now, after beating your head against the wall, that you can't change who they are. Darn!

No one deserves to have a partner with COPD, and no one plans on it. The closest most partners come to being prepared to deal with their spouse's illness is when they are forced to agree with the "in sickness or in health" clause in the marriage contract. It is not quite appropriate to pause during that part of the ceremony to ask for time to think it over—it raises suspicion. Regardless of their disposition and eventual reaction to your COPD, this journey with them (or without them) will have to start with you telling them that you have COPD, which in many cases they already suspect.

Telling Your Partner You Have COPD
Choose the right moment to have this serious talk. Timing is everything. Don't initiate the discussion when you know that time is limited, such as when one of you has to leave in ten minutes for an appointment, are distracted, driving a car, etc.

How you begin the conversation is important. Try to avoid telling your partner while you are angry or doing your best not to burst into tears. Be direct, clear, and don't beat around the bush. Consider starting the conversation with something as straightforward and simple as, "I want to share with you what I learned at the doctor's office today…" I'm not saying that sharing your emotions with your partner is unproductive; just don't let your emotions become the focal point when you first tell him or her. Telling your partner that you have COPD is enough with which to deal! If you approach your partner attuned to his or her feelings, you'll do well.

In some cases, you can almost anticipate the reaction—that's good. By anticipating our partners' reaction, we are better prepared to handle it. If they are going to say, "I told you that you'd get emphysema," or some other dispassionate response, be prepared to bring the discussion back to where it needs to be. If you can't do that, don't let them hook you into their agenda, and don't buy into their negative reaction. Continuing the conversation might do more harm than good. It is better just to let them know you need to put the discussion to rest for a bit (just don't blame them out loud for the delay). Remember that if you catch them off guard, their reaction might be more defensive than empathetic. That's human nature; accept it and move on.

Be also aware that your initial "news" or "discussion" is just that— only the beginning, hopefully, of an ongoing conversation. The purpose is to share the important news so that both of you can prepare to face it together. Don't try to accomplish too much too soon.

If your spouse refuses to deal with your illness and treats it like it is just your problem, you are on very shaky ground. I dare say your relationship problem has little to do with your illness. With the advances in criminal forensics, it no longer pays to try to knock them off. Besides, prison cells can get a bit too stuffy for someone with COPD. You'll have to be more creative.

If you don't have a spouse to contend with or get support from and are doing it alone or relatively alone, you need to take a close look at your support system and think ahead. Be creative and plan things out as best and as carefully as you can. Being alone is not always a disadvantage.

Differences Between Men and Women with COPD

Yes, I hate generalizations as much as the next guy because there are just too many exceptions to the rules, and generalizing slides into stereotyping—something better left to stand-up comedians. Apologies and political correctness aside, spouses might handle your illness differently depending on whether you are a man or woman with COPD.

The Roles We Play

Historically, and in most cultures, women have been prepared or preprogrammed to take care of family and therefore often have some advantages and disadvantages when it comes to having a spouse with COPD. I don't need to point out that traditional roles are changing, so stop rolling your eyes! Whereas men will more likely take care of the "tasks" involved, women will more likely approach their spouse's needs due to their illness on a more emotional level and attend to such things as comfort. Some men simply have a hard time attending to the tasks traditionally "assigned" to women for fear of…I'm not sure…failure, maybe, or a sexual identity meltdown, perhaps?

Emotional Needs and Communicating

Unlike men, women usually want to hear more from their spouse; they want to be told they are important, appreciated, and loved. As an extreme example, if a man takes out the garbage, he can tell he did a good job because the odor is gone. If a woman takes out the garbage, she wants to know her efforts made the living space more comfortable due to the lack of odor, and that her efforts are appreciated because of the care and willingness that was behind the activity—it was an expression of love.

There are differences between men and women not only in regard to the gender of the person with COPD, but also the gender of their mate—assuming one's mate will assume at least some caretaking responsibility. Consequently, there really seems to be two sets of rules! Because our mates didn't come with an owner's manual explaining how they operate under stress, we'll have to use our generic owner's manuals—one for when a man has COPD and one for when a woman has COPD. You'll notice that most people are a combination of qualities from each anyway. Readers in nontraditional relations should read both and apply what fits best. It is also important to point out that when people are sick, regardless of gender, many may have a much lower threshold for annoyances, small problems, noises, or even minor interruptions. Caretakers, regardless of gender, always need to be aware of this when trying to help their partner cope with COPD.

When Men Have COPD

It is interesting to note that women often characterize men as (1) being big babies when they are sick, and/or (2) not acknowledging or talking about their feelings. How can one be a big baby and yet not express feelings? Is this a rather large mute big Baby-Huey some women have in their minds? Actually, these two stereotypical attributes are not in conflict. Many men, when sick, want to be nurtured (and by that I mean taken care of, not petted)! Why the heck shouldn't men want this? Yes, men want their spouses to know they are feeling miserable and want them to do whatever they can to alleviate their discomfort. However, they usually like to accomplish this in as few words as possible. They want to elicit action, not discussion. This form of communication is not to be misinterpreted as disrespect or rejection.

As the disease progresses, the man will probably rely more upon his wife. The man with COPD needs to verbalize what he needs and, equally important, what he don't need. Good communication is a must, and a man with COPD is encouraged to communicate openly and not rely upon his spouse's psychic abilities. If he is smart, he'll help her to feel proud of what she is doing; acknowledge her sacrifices, perseverance, and devotion. Bragging about her to others and having it come back to her will be the start of a very good day indeed!

As the man becomes more SOB, he will experience the eroding of his ability to help with the more physically demanding chores. It is as frustrating as hell! I can't overemphasize this. It is downright humiliating for some men to watch their wives battle to complete physically difficult tasks he was once able to "knock off" with little effort. It is difficult to watch a woman struggle, especially if the tasks are done in an incorrect manner (which is inevitable given the variety of new things they might have to learn). Instructing or correcting them, however, is often heard as criticism, and no one likes to hear criticism or likes to take orders, especially under these circumstances! If this occurs repeatedly, it may put a big strain on the relationship; after all, one partner is trying very hard and feels unappreciated and inept, while the other partner feels guilty and feels as if his advice, as well as himself, is devalued. Don't go there!

Eventually, the list of "duties" and "chores" slowly shift from the "his" list to the "hers" list as the disease progresses. If the man with COPD can pick up some of the things on the "hers' list, that's great. It could be things as simple as paying the bills, slicing vegetables at the table, or even loading the dishwasher. Take time to think through all of the chores to see if the man with COPD can handle them (or parts of them) that require less physical energy. When COPD hits home, it's time to think of chores as not belonging to any gender or role—it is too late for that.

Men with COPD need to be aware of the heightened emotional impact this illness has on their spouses. More often than not, the man is or was the primary provider, and, although things are changing, financial and retirement planning, insurance, maintenance contacts, etc., are often left to him. Men have the responsibility to teach their spouses everything they need to know about their financial and other affairs in order for them to live independently if the man dies first. If your wife is not familiar with some things, teach her what she needs to know. Don't procrastinate; both of you will be more prepared to face the future and thus feel better about it.

Having COPD and helping someone with COPD are both stressful. Do not allow COPD and the frustrations that accompany it to erode your relationship. Both partners should acknowledge out loud that they are aware they are in a frustrating situation and agree not take it out on the other. Because both will inevitably slip, keep the communication open and periodically discuss how it is going and how to make it better. Don't forget the importance of apologies.

Being dependent upon someone is difficult, and it is not unusual for men to refuse help from anyone other than their wives. Although this might be a bit flattering to the wife initially in some strange way, it wears thin very quickly. It is usually a dignity issue. Men need to swallow their pride and, if needed, let others help. It is like jumping into a cold pool; once the initial plunge is taken, the worst is over, and shortly after it is not as uncomfortable as one thought.

When the Woman Has COPD

Most people believe women are prepared to be better caregivers than men. Perhaps they have a point, at least statistically, but I've seen many men who have spouses with COPD who take to the caretaker role surprising well, and some of them have been very *macho*. This may be, in part, because much of the caretaking required is protective and physical in nature. Early in the disease, it is a bit easier because the help that is needed usually involves the more strenuous tasks that the man has been pretty much been doing all along. However, as the disease progresses, the number of chores slowly move from the "her" list to the "his" list until the "his" list includes making meals, shopping, not forgetting to add the fabric softener, and simple things like getting up to get a drink. The switching of items on the "his" and "her" lists is often so gradual that it becomes a smooth transition, mainly because skills are picked up slowly.

One of the common problems women with COPD have when their spouses begin to do house chores is accepting the standards of what their spouses consider clean, timely, well organized or well prepared. Messes may sit around longer, the corners might not be clean, and the cooking might not have the finesse that is desired, but that is a small tradeoff. If women with COPD get significant help from their spouses, it might be high time to relax, realign expectations, and be thankful…very, very thankful!

Men have the reputation of being less able to provide purely emotional support, such as offering reassuring words, lending their shoulder, or understanding the emotional needs caused by trying to adjust to this disease. Women must remember that action speaks louder than words. If he is still with you, he cares.

Unfortunately, some men just don't "get it," and taking over any of the household chores is just not going to happen. They see themselves as protectors, not nurturers, and so they lack any interest or even willingness to pick up more responsibilities. Pressure should shift from trying to get him to help out around the house, to appealing to his protective nature; he can go hunting for a helper to do the chores, or, if necessary, figure out a way to earn the extra money to hire one.

Taking Care of the Caretaker

Who is taking care of the caregiver? There are a couple of things both men and women with COPD can do to support their spouses. The first priority is to ensure that their spouse isn't trading off activities that enrich their lives by having to do the menial chores or having to always stay near their spouse's side. It is not uncommon for someone with COPD to fear being left alone, even for short periods. Those of us with COPD need to make sure our spouses have sufficient quality time away from us. It will help them not only cope with the present, but also help prepare them for the possibility that they will one day be alone without a partner.

Special Problems: Ignoring, Anger, and Smothering

On occasion, people with COPD encounter special problems with their partners as a result, at least in part, of their declining health. It is especially hard to deal with serious relationship problems when you are sick. Most of the problems in relationships that are related to a partner having COPD tend to fall into one of three categories.

Ignoring

Yes, there is always a chance that once you have COPD, your partner will ignore you and your needs. Being ignored is being rejected, and most of us have a hard time with rejection. The ignoring can range from aloofness to a total disinterest in the well-being of the person with COPD. If the ignoring spouse is dealing with his or her own serious health problems, it is understandable. It is still time to join forces.

If we are being ignored or rejected and our partners suggest that our illness and the problems accompanying it are not their responsibility, they probably feel they deserve a seat on a lifeboat. Their lifeboat might be spending as much time out of the home as possible or glued to the sofa in front of the TV three feet from where you spend most of your time. They may even suggest that the person with COPD is faking their inabilities or that it is "all in their head." You can invite them for a dose of reality by joining you during your next doctor's appointment, but don't place any bets on success. Save your money for the casino, where the odds are better.

I think it is fair to say that if you are being ignored, it is not a strong marriage, and if it wasn't for the COPD, something else would have knocked the partnership off its track.

If a respectable level of communication and sufficient caring still remain, it might be beneficial for you to focus on the needs of your spouse. What does he or she need to make the best of it? Again, this is a long shot.

Often, the best approach to a marital problem is to lay it out on the table, preferably with professional help. However, we all know that someone who wants out of a relationship will refuse to participate in any form of counseling or therapy. He or she thinks of counseling as being like one of those glue traps available to catch mice. If you approach the suggestion of getting professional counseling as a way to "help us to decide if we want to go on together or not," you will have a better chance of success than selling it as a way to "work things out."

Anger and Resentment

It is not uncommon for the spouse of someone with COPD to be angry about the illness; however, there is a big difference between being angry at the situation and being angry at you, the person with COPD! The anger may be just a passing stage in coming to terms with your illness, but if doesn't pass, you have a problem. It is easy and even tempting for you to buy into their anger, so be careful. Don't feed off their anger and make matters worse.

If you are a target of your spouse's anger, you neither want to increase their anger nor ignore it, so there are very few options open to you. If one spouse takes his or her anger out on the other and feels better without having to face any consequences, this only reinforces the behavior, and it will usually get worse. Don't let that happen to you! Anger encourages anger, and if anger is met with anger, it will usually just escalate.

If your spouse consistently expresses anger at you, it must be addressed in a way that minimizes his or her defensiveness and does not put his or her ego on the line. It is best that you acknowledge your partner's anger and acknowledge that you can see your illness is really taking a toll on him or her. Avoid being critical during discussions; this includes avoiding being self-critical. Get your partner to agree with you on as many things as you can. The more your partner agrees with you, even over little things, the closer you both are to exploring some possible resolutions. If your partner suggests it is perhaps time for them to "get the hell out of here," let them know it is one of the options that can be explored. You might as well face it now rather than later.

There are times when anger gets out of control and words turn into action. Physical abuse or threats of physical abuse should not be tolerated under any circumstances. They have to be nipped in the bud. Call the police or try to reach someone at a domestic abuse hotline if threats or abuse occur. Your telephone operator can help you find your local center. Whereas women too often blame themselves for abuse, men often feel it unmanly to report that their wives abuse them. Both are unacceptable excuses. Understandable, yes, but still unacceptable. As hard as those calls are to make, they must be made. You deserve better. We all do.

Smothering

You may find that your spouse is smothering you with attention. If he or she tries to do things for you that you are able to do for yourself, constantly asks how you are doing (often when you momentarily forgot you are SOB), or is afraid to leave you alone, it might feel like he or she is smothering you. Frankly, if you consider the alternatives, this isn't a bad problem to have! It could be that your mate is extremely anxious about losing you and fearful about being left alone and unable to deal with the future on his or her own. It is something you can talk about, and indeed do something about. If this is the case, your job is to build up your partner's ego and truly prepare him or her for the future.

In addition to educating our partners about our illness, what is equally important is for them to start treating themselves as good as they treat us! It is our job to ensure that this happens. Let them know how much it pleases you to know they are having a good time, even if it is enjoying activities without you. Encourage them to do things with others and to enjoy life. Encouraging them to enjoy life without you is a one of the greatest gifts you can give.

Sex and Intimacy

You don't have to let COPD destroy your sexual life and intimacy. If you have COPD, the sexuality that often accompanies intimacy might need to be toned down a bit. The trapeze set above the bed might need to be lowered, but it does not need to be taken down. The mate with COPD will usually have to move a bit more slowly or take a more passive physical position, but sexual activity might be better for you than half of the meds you are on! If your sex life has become routine, as is often the case, and it has nothing to do with COPD, your routine might need to be modified (okay, spiced up), and this will require that you talk about sex and physical pleasure with your mate. If you are on O2, you can adjust your O2 flow according to your doctor's instruction. Ask your doctor how far up you can set your O2 flow for sex. Then, just for fun, ask your doctor if that setting is for regular sex or wild sex. If you don't get a laugh, get a new doctor.

Beyond Spouses

We can see the havoc that COPD can create in partnerships, but what is going on with mates is only part of the picture. Other family members are also reacting, and in some cases they might need to provide some of the care at some point. Families can be complex to understand, yet they are often the ones who are there for us in our time of need—or at least that's what we were led to believe.

Chapter 22

FAMILIES OF PEOPLE WITH COPD

Families are like fudge—mostly sweet with a few nuts.
~Author Unknown

If you scratch below the surface of family life, you will usually find more than one individual who should, for the sake of humanity, be confined to the family's closet and never mentioned. I had eight siblings; we didn't have enough closets. Three of us, plus my mother, has or had COPD. Members of your family can be your greatest allies or cause you the deepest pain. But just as we start thinking of what our needs might be down the road, so do many of our family members. It might scare the pants off of some. Eventually, the whole of your family might be somewhat affected by COPD.

Parents and Children

COPD can hit a parent and the family will have to deal with it. COPD can even hit a child and the parent(s) will have to deal with it! Of course, this often occurs when the children are adults and are busy building their own lives. If you are the parent with COPD, your spouse and children are usually the first ones you expect to help you. The expectation can feel like a pressure and an obligation—because it is!

Many families will accept this obligation and try to adjust to it. They'll try their best to balance the many demands placed upon them and make decisions with which they can live. At first, they'll probably try to help out a bit, such as doing the shopping and cleaning. Some members simply can't help, and if it is a larger family, it may develop into sibling rivalries as some members shirk their responsibility knowing that there are others to pick up the slack. There might come a point, however, when the person withCOPD is unable to manage on his or her own. This most often occurs when the COPDer lives alone because his or her spouse is deceased.

Moving in with a Child

In many cases parents will feel totally comfortable with their children taking care of them; it is expected and understood in some families that the children were raised to accept this responsibility when the time comes. This ideal situation does not always exist, however. Children might have other ideas and are often torn between helping to take care of a parent and other demands. One of the most important factors to consider is the in-laws' willingness to extend their home to the mother-in-law or father-in-law with COPD. Understandably, there is often ambivalence or conflict about having to make a decision to invite a parent to move in, and children are torn in different directions. The COPDer is not exempt from feeling conflicted. On one hand, we need and want help, and on the other hand, we don't want to be a burden. It is not unusual for *all sides* to think they'll be screwed regardless of their choice! They are not happy campers. This can be a problem, a big problem!

If you are thinking of moving in with a son or daughter or having an adult child move in with you, here are some things *everyone involved* must consider:

- Who is the primary caregiver, and how good is he or she *really* going to be at it, both skillwise and attitudewise?

- What is the role of the in-law, and how comfortable is he or she with any potential arrangement?

- Is the relationship between the COPDer and caregiver strong enough to endure the frustrations that will occur?

- Are all involved willing to accept the possibility that it might not work out and still remain on good terms?

- How will this affect the caregiver and his or her family, and what might be the consequences each family member must face??

- What is a reasonable commitment of time in months or years?

- What is the physical layout of the house, and will it be comfortable over the agreed-upon term?

- Are there stairs involved, and how might you deal with stairs or other mobility issues over time?

- How involved with the family will the COPDer be? Will he or she be isolated? Will the family have time alone?

- Will the family be open to the COPDer's friends and visitors?

- Who will run errands to pick up meds and such?

- How will the COPDer get to the doctor and other appointments, or will there be a need to change physicians because of the move?

- Will there be opportunities for the COPDer to socialize, get out, and buy a bottle of scotch?

- Is there the physical room and opportunities for the COPDer to engage in hobbies?

- What are the financial arrangements? What is fair, and will all concerned agree *before* moving in? Spell it out with fine detail. There should be no surprises, and although it is really pushing the envelope, you might want to put it in writing. Address any "cost adjustments" that might be required, such as extra electrical costs due to using a concentrator. Will a backup electric generator be needed? Are "caretaker tax credits" available to the family?

- What happens to one's physical possessions? How much can the COPDer bring with him or her?

- What are the "house rules?"

- How far it is from the nearest casino and how will the COPDer get there?

- How do all the "personalities" get along? Do you see any potential problems?

- What can other children, friends or relatives do to pitch in to help the person who has accepted the caretaker responsibilities? Can others pitch in to help with such things as arranging medical services, shopping, transportation to social events, taking care of their laundry, etc?

- Are there built-in opportunities for family members to get a break? Are they expected to be available 24/7 and 365? Caregivers need small breaks and big breaks. How can this be arranged? Can the COPDer vacation or join others for vacations or get away for a season? Are there little breaks built in, such as weekly or monthly opportunities?

- Are backup and emergency plans available in the event the primary caretaker is indisposed?

- How much "care" is expected? Look down the road and anticipate needs in advance (but don't get carried away). Is the caretaker willing and able to assist with such things as bathing and help with a wheelchair?

- Can a trial period be agreed to? It always wise to test it out with a trial period to get a better sense of what it might be like before anyone makes a serious long-term commitment. Remember, everyone is on his or her best behavior during trial periods.

- Can you prearrange opportunities to talk about how it is going so that no one has to let annoying little things build up?

- After the trial period, can all agree to a "no fault" decision regarding moving in or not, where all involved can honestly agree that no one needs to justify why they've made their decision?

- Should you consult with an elder-care attorney regarding future plans, particularly financial and estate planning? Consider discussing "personal care contracts" with the attorney. Personal care contracts, very briefly, allows the person with COPD to pay for his or her care by a relative in a manner that does not compromise the COPDer's future Medicaid eligibility.

- What are other possible alternative living arrangements besides the COPDer moving in?

Avoid "Open-Ended" Agreements

It is highly recommended that no one enter into "open" or "forever" agreements or arrangements. No one, neither the COPDer nor any family member, can predict the future, and unexpected things can and probably will happen! Approach all plans as limited periods of time that, like a lease, can be renewed at the end of each period.

Sharing the Responsibility

The responsibly of taking care of a family member should not rest on any one person's shoulders, if possible. When the member with COPD is unable to live alone and consideration is given to having him or her move in with a son, daughter, or other relative, it might be time for the whole family to sit down and do some "family planning" —and I don't mean deciding how many kids to have!

Often, if responsibility can be shared throughout the family, the person with COPD might be able to spend a few months (or years) with one member before relocating to another member. Yes, it is a nomadic type of existence, but it has some advantages. It can look quite attractive after you've identified the alternatives! What might seem overwhelming for any one person or household to handle can be controllable if enough people are involved and the commitments are of manageable size. Plans such as this require that the family sit down and have a serious discussion. When the words "sharing" and "time-limited commitments" are emphasized, you'll see family members start to think outside the box.

Although family members might be able to "work things out" behind the scenes, therefore saving the COPDer from hearing some of the uncomfortable arguments, once "opportunities" or "possible plans" are identified, be sure the COPDer has all the information and, when possible, makes his or her own decision. If the COPDer is the head of the family, he or she should remain the head of the family. Don't take that away!

If you have COPD, you may feel assaulted repeatedly with losses that are a result of your declining ability to breathe. It takes a toll mentally and emotionally. A large number of us, therefore, experience overwhelming sadness, loneliness, anger, or depression. For some of us, it gets as hard to deal with the emotional consequences of the illness as it does the physical limitations imposed.

Chapter 23

DEALING WITH SADNESS, LONELINESS, AN-GER, AND DEPRESSION

One cannot be deeply responsive to the world without being saddened very often.
~Erich Fromm

It is often hard to be calm, positive, and optimistic while we are being bombarded with the day-to-day struggles that seem to accompany having COPD. Often, problems related to our COPD are piled atop the other struggles we face that may have nothing to do with our disease. It can all get overwhelming. When our feelings are hard to endure, we wonder what, if anything, we can do to make them go away or at least become more bearable. Fortunately, there are some things we can do to help ourselves.

Good and Bad Feelings
We tend to put all of our feelings into one of two categories: "good" or "bad." We've given many different names to "bad" feelings, such as "down," "sad," "hurt," "frightened," "miserable," "crappy," "depressed," etc. Of course, feelings are not really "good" or "bad," they just are. Feelings, like pain, can tell us that things aren't they way they need to be; they signal the need for change. So-called "bad" feelings can also be our reaction to experiencing unmet needs or giving up the hope of doing some of the things we looked forward to. It is normal to feel "bad" after a loss. The loss can be real, such as a loss of a job or a person in our lives. An equally painful sense of loss can also be experienced when the loss is that of a dream or expectation, such as having a healthy retirement, feeling youthful and sexy, etc. When our expectations are shattered, our sense of loss is real and painful. We often make our problem of pain worse in the long haul by numbing ourselves or cutting off our feelings. Things that provide short-term relief can sometimes grow into bigger problems.

Having COPD can bring with it all types of feelings: fear, sadness, loneliness, and even anger. For some of us, our feelings can take the joy out of being alive. They can become so intense and prolonged that they become disabling. It is also important for us to learn to recognize when we need to seek professional help and to be aware of what kind of help is available to us. By understanding our feelings and dealing with some of the uncomfortable ones, we can make living with COPD easier.

Sadness, loneliness, anger, grief, and an illness called depression are all common complaints from people with COPD, so we'll look at each of them:

Sadness

We have all experienced sadness—no doubt great sadness in our lives. Sadness is about losing something, anything; it could be a real loss of something tangible, like one's home, or it could be the loss of an expectation, dream, or belief. Sometimes we get sad just by recalling past events because they remind us of things now gone. Being sad at times is just part of being human, so don't think of it as something unnatural or assume there is anything wrong with feeling sad.

We all deal with sadness and adversity differently. I know people with COPD who have very few problems dealing with their illness, and I also know others who are miserable. Being told to "keep your chin up," "pull yourself up by your bootstraps," or "your glass is half full," although well-intentioned, is useless and annoying. Ignore people who say such things, and if you can, let the air out of their tires.

Medical Causes

Chronic sadness or symptoms of depression (detailed later) can have medical origins such as illnesses, medications, hormonal or metabolic problems, or even a seasonal affective disorder. If you are not feeling up to par, it is always important to consider possible medical causes, especially if symptoms are significant. Let your doctor know what is going on, and ask him or her to rule out underlying medical causes for your distress.

Ten Common Causes of Sadness and How to Deal with Them

If you are cheerfully whistling and believe your cup is half full, you should avoid reading the following. It will irritate you. Instead, go check your tires. Here is a list of losses common to people with COPD and some thoughts on how to deal with them. Remember, however, we are all at different.

1. **Decrease in Attractiveness**
   Here's the Deal: Sure, we pant, but it is not the type of panting that people find attractive. Don't give up. Make yourself as attractive as you can and remind yourself that beauty is only skin deep. Sometimes, people who feel less attractive spend less rather than more time with their appearance, so spend extra time enhancing your appearance. Allow your personality and attitude to attract people. Fake it if you have to. If it works, it just might become automatic and natural.

2. **Less Sex**
   Here's the Deal: Although similar to "attractiveness" above, please know that you don't have to give up sex—just slow it down. Don't pretend with me that in the past you didn't land on your feet after sex and expect the judges to hold up their score cards! You may need to talk to your partner about limitations and use those positions you used to complain were the "lazy" way out. Don't forget to think sexy and introduce some novelties and incentives. Leaving cash on the nightstand is not considered a proper incentive.

3. **Missing Work**
   Here's the Deal: Replace some of the meaningful activities you lost when you retired. It is important to engage in performing significant and satisfying activities, which include volunteering, hobbies, and learning new things. If you can, include others in these activities so you also get the reward of social contacts.

4. **Less Income**
   Here's the Deal: If you are receiving Social Security income or Social Security Disability Income, you are allowed to earn up to a specific amount without it affecting your benefits. Be sure you are maximizing your benefits by visiting www.benefitscheckup.org. Also, there are many good suggestions on how to economize at www.cheapskatemonthly.com.

5. **Social Contacts**
   Here's the Deal: It really is hard to maintain social contacts when your mobility and energy are zapped due to COPD, and it is very easy to give up trying to be social. Don't give up. You just have to keep working at it. Use the Internet to meet people.

6. **Decreased Independence**
   Here's the Deal: There isn't much you can do about being dependent upon others; however, you can stop feeling guilty about it. Although you can't change being dependent upon others, you can make their support easier by being pleasant to be with. Your good humor, sincere appreciation, love, and concern for their well-being can be valuable payoffs. People actually volunteer to help others just to be appreciated, so don't think of it as a one-way street!

7. **Loss of Control**
   Here's the Deal: If you can't control something, let it go!

8. **Dreams and Plans**
   Here's the Deal: It is okay to shed a tear when you give up dreams. It is important to say goodbye to them or to modify them. You still may be able to live your dreams, but in a modified or scaled-down version. Realize it is not the particular site or location that you will miss, such as seeing the Grand Canyon, for example; it is the anticipation of your reaction to those sites that you will miss! You wanted the thrill and awe. Please realize that the thrill and awe are within you and not the rocks and canyons! If you desire to be speechless and in awe of the Great Master's work, be aware there are creations in your own back yard that can also be awe-inspiring if you let them. Peering under a microscope can be as amazing as looking through a pair of binoculars—if you let it. I find Milton's words always inspiring when I'm feeling cheated. I believe he really "got it!"

   > To see a world in a grain of sand,
   > And a heaven in a wild flower,
   > Hold infinity in the palm of your hand,
   > And eternity in an hour.

9. **Low Self-esteem**
   Here's the Deal: You need to keep feeling good about your-self, and that means not feeling guilty for your COPD and what it does to you and others around you.

   As a matter of fact, cut off all mind chatter related to nega-tive evaluations of yourself. Stop those endless tapes of nega-tive thoughts in your head. Hit the stop button every time you catch yourself thinking negatively about yourself. Repeat hit-ting that button every time the negative chatter starts. You'll be surprised at how often you have to hit the stop button, but eventually your patience will pay off. Also, if you can, add val-ue to those around you by helping them in any way you can. If there is nothing you can do, you can always take on the hard-est task, and that is to demonstrate to those around you how to deal with adversity, so they have a role model when and if their time comes.

   Much of how we feel comes from the regard others have towards us, so stay away from people who tear you down.

   You can also feel better about yourself for your accom-plishments. Set achievable small goals. Eventually, you be able to take on larger projects that.

Loneliness

Loneliness is sadness, a special type of sadness, that includes a sense of emptiness and isolation, and a feeling that you crave company or companionship. Wanting desperately to be with someone can be ex-ceedingly uncomfortable. Loneliness is like a toothache in your heart. Some people find comfort and safety in being alone, and others find it uncomfortable—some to the point where being alone is unbear-able. Aloneness is different than loneliness. Aloneness is a state of be-ing; it is neither good nor bad—it just is. It is important to know that being alone does not have to result in feeling lonely.

Loneliness can come either from not having enough meaning-ful connections or from having connections to others that are not working properly, not unlike being plugged in without the electricity turned on. Loneliness, like sadness, is part of life, and most of us have found our way out of bouts of loneliness. Loneliness can be a passing feeling on a Saturday night as you sit alone, or it can be an almost constant, unbearable, empty feeling that constantly haunts you. Due to our illness, we are often forced to spend more time alone than we would like. Time alone gives us a lot of time to reflect upon our lives. Some people find this difficult, but there are a few things you can do:

1. **Get Out and Socialize More or Invite People Over**
   A surprising number of people complain of loneliness, but when you ask them what they've done about it, they are rather mute and change the subject. Once you establish contact with someone, make their time enjoyable. They are not going to come back if your time with them is spent complaining or dealing with sadness.

2. **Revitalize Your Current Contacts**
   Take stock of the social outlets, friends, relatives you do have, and work on making those relationships deeper and more meaningful.

3. **Learn to Be Alone**
   Some people equate being alone to being lonely; they are different! The solution, obviously, is learning to feel okay about being alone; this requires both keeping yourself entertained as well as not experiencing anxiety over being alone. Discover what good company you can be to yourself. Consider pursuing some hobbies that you find entertaining so that your "solitude" is pleasurable instead of uncomfortable. If you feel anxious when alone, relaxation exercises or meditation can be very useful.

4. **Become Aware of Internal Dialogues**
   Loneliness, according to some experts, is simply a self-esteem problem. Become aware of the mind chatter and begin to change it so that it is more positive; let that internal dialogue not be so stingy with praise throughout the day. Compliment yourself on what you were able to do, and let yourself feel proud of your many small accomplishments throughout the day.

Anger and Irritability

Anger is the natural response to a perceived frustration or threat to our well-being. It can be a precursor to aggression. Anger can range from being annoyed to intense rage. Many of us have a "low-grade" anger—others call us "crabby" (or worse). Anger has some interesting qualities. Understanding those qualities can help us deal with our anger more effectively:

Anger is Physiological and Psychological

You can tell when someone is angry. You can see it in their body tension, alertness, language, physical appearance, and even movement; when someone is angry, physiological things happen inside of the body, such as increased heart rate, increased blood pressure, and increased adrenaline. It is unhealthy both physically and mentally.

Anger Can be a Result of a Threat Either Real, Anticipated, or Imagined

We can react to threats to our well-being regardless of whether the threat is a real physical threat or something we "think" might eventually harm us.

Anger Can Be at Oneself

Anger probably came about as a way to get us ready to defend ourselves from external threats or overcome obstacles. Due to our large brain and ability to reason, we sometimes conclude that our own actions are a threat to our well-being and we can become angry at ourselves. Anger can also be a mask for sadness and loneliness.

Anger Can Have Many Sources

Not only do we get angry in preparation to protect ourselves, avoid pain, or remove barriers, we can become angry over small things that hurt our feelings, especially those things we think of as assaults to our self-image or ego. Worse, we can store them up. We sometimes store them under our mental list of "injustices." Try to avoid being an "injustice collector."

Dealing with Anger

Actually, dealing with anger is very difficult. Dealing with anger directly through violence towards others is usually unlawful, so put those dueling pistols away. You can always try to deal with your anger by using passive-aggressive approaches (inactions such as the ever-popular silent treatment), but they seldom work and just annoy others.

Being irritable and crabby is no way to live. It is hard to feel joy when you are feeling irritable or crabby. Nevertheless, we all have bad days and bad periods. Being angry or irritable on occasion is nothing over which to be concerned; sometimes, in fact, it is just part of the healing process when grieving over a loss in one's life. Just don't let it become a disposition!

So what do you do with this anger? Because you have to meet the threat head on but without fists, use reasoning and understanding to replace physical violence. The process, however, depends on the source of the anger:

If a situation or condition is the cause of your anger (frustration):

Your best recourse is to try to solve the problem causing the anger; get help if you need help to solve it. Find ways around the problem, try to lessen it, resolve it, or avoid it. If you can't change it, you have no other option other than to accept it.

If a person and/or their actions is the cause of your anger:

Talk it out. Try this approach:

1. Don't be angry when you talk to them.

2. Remind yourself that we all make mistakes and the person you are talking to has his or her own issues.

3. Don't use the opportunity to try to make the person feel bad or guilty.

4. Don't focus on what the person did "wrong" but instead focus *briefly* on describing how you felt in response to what he or she said or did.

5. Avoid name calling, being critical, or coming across as judgmental.

6. Ask for what you want. Ask the person to approach you or the problem In a different manner, and make your request specific. Start your request with such phrases as:

    a. If this happens again, I'd like to ask you to…

    b. I'd like it if you could…

    c. I want…

    d. Please…

    Watch your tone of voice, as even the above can come across as sarcastic! And don't use the word "should"!

7. Be aware that even if you don't get the response you would like, the simple act of talking to the person about the problem will sometimes result in your anger dissipating. Also, it might take time for the person to digest your conversation (or save face).

8. If the above doesn't work, you can make a conscious decision to let bygones be bygones and actually forgive the person as you would hope you would be forgiven—hmmm, this reminds me of a prayer I once heard!

If You Are Angry at Yourself
Do you sometimes think you "ought to have, could have, should have, would have," etc., done things differently? Do you blame it on your stubbornness, stupidity, rebellion, greed, indifference, or some other negative motive about which you should feel ashamed? Atone, apologize, stand on your head, or do whatever you need to do to bring this to an end. Simply forgiving yourself for being human and making mistakes is the most direct route. If the angry feelings are associated with thoughts, change those negative thoughts as they pop up and replace them with positive ones. If you find it hard to forgive yourself, start first by forgiving others. Some people believe this is a prerequisite to forgiving yourself.

Depression

Overview of Depression

Depression feels like great sadness and great loneliness are teaming up together, perhaps inviting in some anger and punching the spirit out of you. The words "helpless" and "hopeless" are often used to describe the state of mind of someone in the midst of a depression, but the words don't always do it justice. The experience is almost beyond words. Depression is not only about feelings; depression also affects our bodies and our thinking. Brain scans are able to show how it affects certain parts of our brains; depression is a *real physical illness* and *not* the result of some moral or character weakness.

One of the biggest misunderstandings about depression is that it is an attitude problem and that you can do something about it if you just change your attitude! Depression is an illness.

The Causes of Depression

There are many theories of the origin of depression, but regardless of theories, we do know genetics can play a significant part of it. One of the most popular views of depression is that it comes about due to loss (or an accumulation of losses) that one cannot overcome. When depressed, just about everything seems to be dulled or turned down: perception, energy, meaningfulness, social connections, thinking, hope, the feeling or belief that you can make changes to your life, your value in this world, and, one of the most harmful in my opinion, the ability to enjoy your life, even in little bits here and there. Unfortunately, fear and anxiety are not always dampened, and they can become intense while you're depressed.

Depression seems to run in families, but it requires something in our lives to trigger it. Unfortunately, you can develop depression even if you have no family history of it. What we think of and define as depression is probably not just one illness but a group of closely related illnesses; it is all a rather murky area. Symptoms can vary among individuals, sometimes dramatically. The experience of depression can be the result of many different things other than psychological triggers; it can also come from medications, illnesses such as mononucleosis, thyroid problems, chemical imbalances, seasonal affective disorder, or other medical conditions. It is for this reason that *a full medical evaluation absolutely should take place to rule out other identifiable causes before we conclude we are experiencing the type of depression we are discussing.*

Diagnosis of Depression

The good news is that depression is treatable, but it first has to be properly diagnosed. There are medications available that can correct some of the brain chemistry that has changed as part of the depression. If other medical causes for depression have been ruled out, the person needs to be evaluated to determine what type of features or symptoms the depression has, because there are different types or manifestations of depression. The symptoms of depression vary widely and include the following; however, you do not have to have all or even most of the symptoms:

Symptoms

*   Feelings of helplessness, hopelessness, or bleakness

*   Persistent sadness or sense of emptiness

*   Feeling or believing that nothing will get better

*   Feelings of worthlessness or guilt

*   Difficulty concentrating, remembering things, or making decisions

*   Agitation, restlessness, or irritability nearly every day

*   Fatigue or sluggishness

*   Loss of interest in usual activities, hobbies, social activities, or sex

*   Withdrawal from social situations, family, or friends

*   Changes in appetite or weight gain or loss

*   Changes in sleep patterns, either insomnia or oversleeping

*   Aches and pains: headaches, backaches, digestive problems, or aching joints

*   Thoughts of death, suicide plans, or attempts

If you have *any* symptoms of depression, you should seek help. If your symptoms include hallucinations or suicidal thoughts, you should seek medical attention *immediately*. Call your doctor right away or get emergency room treatment. You deserve help even if you don't feel like you do. The day will come that you will be extremely thankful you got help.

Types of Depression

Many mental health professionals often break depression down into two types:

1. Reactive depression: This is a prolonged grieving response to known, identifiable losses, usually near the onset of symptoms. Reactive depression is thought to be shorter lived.

2. Major depression (or clinical depression): Major depression often originates in childhood and is lifelong or not attributable to specific identifiable recent losses. People can be mildly depressed and spend their whole lives with an underlying depression, or overwhelmed by their depression and unable to function.

Depression is not uncommon, especially for people with COPD. It seems that you barely adjust or recover from one thing and you are hit with another. No wonder between 25% and 50% of us report being depressed. COPD has a peculiar proclivity to bombard us over a long period of time with losses, and this can wear us down. It seems there is always one more straw waiting in the wings to break our backs. It is important to be reminded that there are a large number of us who deal quite well with our COPD and do not get depressed. Being depressed is not inevitable if you have COPD, but treatable if you do have it.

Treatment

A self-help book is simply not a good enough treatment for depression! If you are diagnosed with depression, it is important you get proper care. There are two main types of treatment, medication and psychotherapy.

Medication

There are many drugs available to treat depression. Getting the right medication and getting it in the right dose can be tricky, so be patient. A psychiatrist will have more experience with medications for depression than most other doctors. Because some take time to "kick in," they can sometimes help you temporarily with other medications. Primary care physicians and pulmonologists frequently prescribe antidepressants.

Talk Therapy
Talk therapy can be very effective in treating depression and is believed by therapists to be one of the most treatable conditions. The combination of medication and talk therapy might be the most potent way to deal with your depression. It worked for me.

Finding a Qualified Psychotherapist
You not only want to find someone well qualified, you also want to find someone with whom you are comfortable. This might require checking out a couple or more potential therapists. You can locate a therapist in one in the following ways:

- Ask your physician for a referral.

- Check with family or friends for a referral. Ask what they like and do not like about the therapist.

- Check with your church, synagogue, mosque, or religious center; however, be sure that the person to whom you are referred is properly credentialed—something occasionally overlooked by some religious organizations.

- Call or visit the Web site of your local hospital for a psychiatrist listed with the hospital, or use the hospital's referral service.

- Check the phone book or use the Internet to find a local mental health center or community health association. Some offer fees on a sliding scale.

- Call the American Psychological Association's consumer information help line at 800-964-2000 for referral information to a licensed psychologist.

- Visit the National Association of Social Workers at www.socialworkers.org/nasw which allows you to find certified social workers in your area who are experienced specifically with depression

Dealing with COPD is not easy and indeed, it is not even a one-shot deal; it is ongoing. If you talk to others with COPD, you will find that although some of us experience sadness, loneliness, depression, or anger, a large number of us are faced with equally challenging reactions: fear, anxiety, panic, and phobias! Some of us even have a combination.

Chapter 24

DEALING WITH FEAR, ANXIETY, PANIC, AND PHOBIAS

Fear is faith that it won't work out.
~Sister Mary Tricky

Fear, phobias, anxiety, and panic are all related; they are like conspiring cousins. Anxiety and panic are common problems with us COPDers. Some of us are claustrophobic, too! As our COPD progresses, it too often feels like we are living a bit too close to the edge, and that is very hard to endure over a long period of time. Before we can begin to deal with the problems of fear, anxiety, panic, and phobias, we first need to understand them. In a way, they are all too much of a good thing; they are natural and even protective responses that have gone a bit awry. Fear, anxiety, panic, and even the origins of phobias are natural ways to protect ourselves, and they work fine as long as they don't go overboard, get carried away, or have a life of their own. If they do, they end up working against us.

As animals, our number one priority is to protect ourselves so we're around to procreate. No, I'm not going to talk about sex here, so don't get too excited! Back in the good old days, when we humans were running through the forests grunting, stabbing mammoths, and defending ourselves against saber-tooth tigers, we needed to be prepared to fight for our lives or run for our lives. This is the well-known "fight or flight" response. It worked well. We're still around.

Fear
Fear increases alertness and results in other physical changes to get our bodies and muscles ready for either the serious workout that might be required to defend ourselves or to outrun our adversaries. Hormones like adrenalin are released in our bodies to pump more blood to our muscles to increase their O2 level. We breathe harder to keep the O2 level up also. The fear can also turn into aggression and anger if they are needed to protect ourselves. Fear can arise from a

tangible threat—a real danger you can see, such as a car barreling towards you, or an imagined, anticipated, or unknown source, such as not knowing what lurks around the next corner, being ridiculed, or fear of the outcome of a medical test. Additionally, our imaginations can run wild. We even fear threats to our self-image and prepare ourselves for an assault as if it were a real physical threat. However, in most cases, we neither run nor fight, so we're stuck in a body with the motor racing and are stuck in neutral. This is not only uncomfortable, it is harmful.

Anxiety

Anxiety and fear are very similar. The term "fear" is usually used when the threat is known, such as fearing snakes or catching an illness. The term "anxiety" is usually used when the cause of the fear is unknown, diffuse, or when just about everything triggers a fear response, kind of like a constant worry or constant state of fear. Anxiety can range from a low level, feeling fidgety or jumpy, to a level that is truly overwhelming.

Anxiety often seems to feed anxiety; we become worried about our anxiety, and that makes matters even worse. When you can't figure out the cause of the anxiety you are experiencing, can't escape the disturbing feeling, and can't run away from yourself, you might wonder if you are losing your mind or going off the deep end. Please be assured that if you are experiencing this, you are not going crazy.

If the state of anxiety is prolonged, out of proportion, and becomes a mind-set that affects one's life, it is considered a "generalized anxiety disorder." Feeling edgy, irritable, and tense often affects our digestion, resulting in stomach or bowel problems, including ulcers. It can disrupt or interfere with sleeping, eating, and virtually every aspect of life. It affects us biologically, psychologically, and in our relationships. Anxiety and anxiety disorders can be treated with medications and psychotherapy. Anxiety can also be a part of depression, although the degree of each can vary.

Because anxiety is not just in the head, but also in the body, we require more O2 when anxious. Yes, anxiety can contribute to SOB—the last thing you need if you are SOB! It is a double problem for us because it can become a vicious cycle: anxiety can make you more

SOB, which can make you more anxious…you get the picture! Simply treating anxiety can help some people breathe better.

Panic Attacks and Anxiety Attacks

Panic attacks are often referred to as anxiety attacks; however, one can have serious anxiety attacks (or episodes) that fall short of being full-blown panic attacks. Once you have had an all-out panic attack, you know you've had one!

If you have panic attacks, they probably feel the same as our ancestors' panic when they noticed a hungry saber-tooth tiger with a gleam in his eye licking his chops. Panic is our built-in emergency response system. Panic *demands* that you do something, anything, *immediately*! Frankly, it can feel like you are about to die. Many of us with COPD have bouts of extreme anxiety when we are unable to catch our breath. The fear of not being able to recover our breath can lead to the sensation that we are suffocating to death and can, for darn good reason, cause us to panic.

Some sources say the average panic attack is about 10 minutes, and other experts say most are over within 20 minutes, but they can be longer or shorter. If we have repeated panic attacks, we are labeled as having a "panic disorder." You should feel no more embarrassed by this label than you would if you had a "metabolic disorder."

One of the biggest problems for some people who have panic attacks is that they are often not aware of what triggers their attacks, and therefore they have a hard time avoiding them. Panic and anxiety attacks that seem to come out of nowhere are especially disconcerting, and they often come at the worst possible time—perhaps because that is when we fear having them the most! The mere worry about having one can cause one. If you have panic attacks, even if you don't know what triggers them, you are not insane.

Having COPD and panic attacks is a bad combination. The bad thing about panic attacks is that, by definition, they are the opposite of relaxation, and, as mentioned earlier, they use up more O2—the one thing you need most when you are SOB! Panic can feed upon itself to the point where it is so acute it can cause one to defecate in one's pants. This is the origin of the old saying that something can "scare the shit out of you." Panic attacks can include the following, although you don't have to have all of them to have a panic disorder:

Physical
    Rapid heartbeat and/or chest pain
    Sweating and/or hot flashes and/or chills
    Nausea or abdominal cramping
    Fainting or dizziness
    Headache
    Shortness of breath or hyperventilating
    Shaking or trembling
    Tightness in throat or problem swallowing

Mental
    Sense or fear you are dying
    Absolute terror
    Feeling like you want to run and/or scream

As you can see, the physiological symptoms are quite intense, and the body is taxed to the extreme. This can be dangerous, so *if you think you are having panic attacks and you have not been diagnosed as having them, you must seek medical help immediately to rule out other causes!*

Evaluation and Treatment of Panic and Anxiety
Once a medical evaluation has ruled out serious illnesses or other causes for your panic attacks, such as cardiac, thyroid, or other conditions, and you are diagnosed as having an anxiety or panic disorder, you are ready to consider treatment. Medication as well as talk-therapy, specifically "cognitive behavioral therapy," can help tremendously.

To find a cognitive behavioral therapist in your area, you can contact the National Association of Cognitive Behavioral Therapists at 1-800-853-113 or www.nacbt.org.

Relaxation, Meditation Techniques, and Music
Meditation, in one form or another, is practiced in most, if not all, of the world's major religions. All the religions seem to have their own unique approaches and objectives of meditation. One thing they seem to hold in common is they provide an escape from the type of thinking we all automatically fall into. We benefit by focusing our attention on a fixed point rather than allowing our thoughts to wander at the expense of being in the present. A common component of meditation is to either train or allow the mind

to focus on something other than the thoughts that usually occur. One analogy is that it is like turning the engine off to let it cool down and rest. Fortunately, many of the same benefits of meditations can be achieved by nonreligious meditation techniques. The nonreligious ones are often called "relaxation techniques" or "systematic relaxation." These techniques are an effective way to relax that leads to a number of benefits:

- Stress reduction and relaxation

- Muscle relaxation

- Increased immune response (possibly due to less stress)

- Decreased blood pressure

- Improved blood flow to muscles

- Reduce need for O2

- Reduction of symptoms such as headaches and back pain

- Better energy

- Better concentration

- Better ability to handle problems

There are many techniques, and some specifically ask you to first relax your muscles. Some relaxation techniques skip this and will introduce something to focus on, knowing that once appropriately focused, your body will begin to relax automatically.

1. Choose a good time of the day to start your relaxation. Pick two periods of fifteen minutes each, preferably a few hours before bedtime or eating.

2. Find a suitable location away from all distractions, especially noise.

3. Get into a comfortable position, which for us is usually sitting. If you have to, you can do this lying down, although sitting up is preferred. The purpose is to make the body comfortable without inducing sleep. Avoid slouching, dangling the arms, crossing the legs, etc. Keep your feet flat on the floor and your hands resting on your lap.

4. Focus first on your breathing to find a comfortable, measured pace. Allow yourself time to relax with your eyes closed. Focus upon being comfortable and breathe from the diaphragm. Inhale through the nose and exhale out your mouth if possible; however, it is not required.

5. Start to relax your muscles by working the muscle groups: first start with your toes, then feet, then lower legs, upper legs, stomach, torso, hands, arms, back, and then neck. You can move your neck around a bit very slowly and let it find a comfortable position without dropping forward. Take time with each muscle group and think of it becoming relaxed, heavy, warm, and "dead weight." Eventually, you will learn what relaxation really feels like, and you will be able to do it on command.

6. You now want to focus your mind on something that has a neutral or good association but doesn't provoke much thought or reaction. In religious practices, this would often be called a mantra (a repeated word or phrase). So pick a word or very short phrase. Although religious phrases will work, such as "Jesus is my savior," one might be inclined to start thinking about religious beliefs, etc. Try not to contemplate or get into a deep or particular thought; you are trying to do the opposite, not think, and to relax. Good word choices might be: "comfort," "peace," "one," "nice," etc. This is the same word or phrase you will use each time. You are not going to change the word because the word or phrase, after it is used repeatedly, will become associated with relaxation and will help you relax quickly.

7. You will now repeat this word or short phrase silently to yourself in a slow, comfortable manner.

8. As you repeat this phrase, you will find your mind wandering to other thoughts. This is not bad; just bring your mind back to the word. Do not react to the many times your mind wanders by getting annoyed or upset, because it is a natural process. Simply bring your mind back to the word or phrase. If something happens to distract you, such as a car horn, door slamming, or phone ringing, just accept it without annoyance and simply bring your mind back to the word or phrase. Life happens and it is okay.

9. If you fall asleep, that isn't bad. All it means is that you need sleep. Bring yourself back to your relaxation exercise and back into the more alert position.

10. Keep a clock or watch available to check the time so you can tell when your fifteen minutes are up. Try to put the timepiece in front of you so you don't have to crane or move your neck or grab a pair of glasses to see the time. When you check the time, do so slowly and only open one eye, and only as far open as needed. Absolutely do not set an alarm!

11. When your time is up, stop focusing on your word or phrase. Stay relaxed for a couple of minutes and then slowly open your eyes one at a time. Open and close your eyes as often as you like to make the transition gradual. Then start moving one foot, then the other, etc. Make it an easy adjustment from relaxation into your regular state of mind.

12. Let yourself feel your body and how it feels to be relaxed. Enjoy it. Try to take the relaxation with you once your relaxation period is over. You will often realize how relaxed you've become the moment you stand. Be careful when starting to stand because you muscles might be very relaxed!

13. Get into the habit of making relaxing (or meditation) an important part of your everyday life. The effects are cumulative, and the longer you stay with it, the more you will get from it. If you can't do it twice a day, which is highly preferable, at least do it once.

The great thing about using relaxation techniques is that they work in two ways for us COPDers with anxiety. In addition to the benefits listed above, if you are becoming anxious or are panicked, you can have a seat, close your eyes, and start using your relaxation word with pursed lip breathing and breathing from the diaphragm. Don't forget to relax your shoulders. During your daily relaxation routine, your mind has associated the feeling of relaxation with the word or mantra you repeat, and you will learn to automatically begin to relax upon silently repeating the word. Being able to meet the fear and anxiety with their opposite is a potent way of dealing with anxiety and anxiety attacks.

One of the great proponents of relaxation techniques and the man who coined the phrase "relaxation response" is Herbert Benson, MD. For information about his technique as well as books, tapes, CDs, etc., you can contact the Benson-Henry Institute for Mind Body Medicine at Massachusetts General Hospital at www.massgeneral.org/bhi or call (617) 732-9130.

Visualization Techniques
There are also techniques to help you relax that use visualization, such as focusing on a peaceful, restful scene, often a beach with the patterns of the waves crashing on shore. If you would like, you can substitute a visualization for a word or phrase. There is also a large variety of tapes and CDs available over the Internet and in bookstores to help you learn to relax.

Hypnosis and Self-hypnosis
Hypnosis is simply another similar technique that can induce relaxation. Many of the relaxation tapes that are available are self-hypnosis tapes. Purists, however, often maintain that meditation and hypnosis are opposites.

Refocusing
When feeling anxious, rather than dwelling on it or becoming more acutely aware of your anxiety level increasing and worrying about the increase, try to get your mind away from thinking about it. I play solitaire on the computer, but reading a poem, making a list, or engaging in some other nonphysical activity requiring some concentration can prevent the anxiety from escalating. Anxiety attacks are usually short-lived, and this might help you not only relax a bit but ride it out by distracting yourself.

Breathing Exercises
Calm, measured, and controlled pursed lip breathing (see the chapter on breathing techniques) will also help you to relax. Remember that relaxation is the antidote for anxiety because you can't be anxious and relaxed at the same time. If you can do the controlled breathing along with the above refocusing or relaxation techniques, you will have a very nice combination—one which has saved my tail a good number of times.

Social Support

Talking about your fear and anxiety with someone can help you put it in perspective and might even help you to control it. Also, having someone to call when you are having an acute episode can make all the difference in the world.

Physical Health

Proper diet and exercise can both play a role in helping you deal with stress. Exercise can help you "work off" nervous energy and keep your whole body better prepared to deal with anxiety. Eliminating or cutting back on caffeine and alcohol often helps decrease nervousness or anxiety.

Stress Management

One way (but not the only way) to look at stress management is to consider "stress" to be the difference between demands placed upon you and your resources for dealing with those demands. Hey, if you could handle huge demands you wouldn't have a problem with stress, now would you? Take a serious look at the demands upon you and the resources you have to meet those demands. Do what you need to do to create a workable balance.

Phobias

A phobia is another natural fear response that has taken on a life of its own. By definition, a phobia is an "irrational" fear; however, an irrational fear is only a problem if it interferes in your life. You can be afraid of bananas, for example, but they can easily be avoided—well, unless, of course, you live in Honduras! If you become afraid of open areas or enclosed areas, for example, you are in trouble. It is just too hard for most of us to avoid such places. The phobic reaction can range from mild to outright panic attacks. You can begin to see how these things—fear, anxiety, panic and phobias—are all related.

The term "irrational" often causes some confusion. In some cases yes, the fear can be quite irrational, such as fear of stepping on a crack in the sidewalk, but more often the term "irrational" is used to simply describe a reaction that is way out of proportion or more extreme than what the average person experiences. What is "irrational" is that the fear is way out of proportion to the odds of actually being injured. "Irrational" does not mean "crazy"!

The strange thing about a phobia is that if you turn it on its head, it might be considered hope. I'll explain: If you have a million-in-one chance of winning a lottery and believe in your heart you are actually holding the winning ticket, it is hope and faith. The opposite side of the coin is to believe for sure you will be injured even if the odds are a million-to-one. A phobia is, therefore, nothing of which to be ashamed. It is reverse hope!

Those of us with COPD often develop phobias related to our fear of not being able to breathe. Enclosed spaces such as elevators, MRI machines, long halls without windows, basements, etc., or even the thought of them, can be disturbing.

There is one last very important thing to understand about phobias. It goes back to how our brains are wired. Once the brain starts processing things, be it fear or how to decrease it, the brain can become "hard-wired." Hard wiring means automatically taking a well-worn path in the brain when the switch is hit. A certain thought or exposure to something can trigger the reaction, even if it no longer seems to have anything to do with the original fear. The good news is that if fear can be hard-wired, other responses such as relaxation can also be hard-wired.

Treatment of Phobias

It is hard to treat a phobia yourself. A standard treatment technique is to expose people with a phobia to small increments of the thing that frightens them while they are relaxed. They would approach the phobic object when relaxed, so that they slowly begin to override the panic response and lean a new response. Each treatment would get the person a bit closer to the feared object or activity while being relaxed. The person, in effect, is "desensitized." If you are bothered by fear, anxiety, or phobias, you owe it to yourself to fight them by getting appropriate help. You'll be glad you did.

As much of our fear and anxiety has to do with the future and what the future has in store for us, it is important for us to take as much control over the future as possible. Although some of us will have more control than others, often due to financial assets, long-term care insurance, and other factors, it is important to plan for your future the best you can.

Chapter 25

PLANNING FOR YOUR CONTINUED CARE

If you don't design your own life plan, chances are you'll fall into someone else's plan. And guess what they have planned for you? Not much.
~ Jim Rohn

If we have COPD, we must realize that our needs are going to increase over time. We must also accept that our needs may increase beyond the capabilities of those available to help us. We can perhaps get someone to help us in our homes, or we can move into the home of a son, daughter, friend or relative, or look into a structured living arrangement. Too many of us procrastinate planning for such a future because we believe that somehow doing this will magically buy us more time. It doesn't work.

In order to plan for the future, we first need to know what is available to us outside of our personal resources of family and friends.

Community-Based Services
Community-based services are services provided by local or state organizations to help older and/or disabled adults remain in their homes. They are paid for by local (city or county) funds, state funds, or grants. Services are free or low cost. Because they are local, they vary widely from state to state and area to area within each state, so check out local resources. Some of the services available in selected areas include personal care, transportation services, running errands, case management, telephone reassurance, etc. If you are older, you can locate the services available in your area by visiting the Eldercare Locator at www.eldercare.gov or calling (800) 677-1116. You can also check to see if the Meals on Wheels Program (www.mowaa.org or 703-548-5558) is available in your community.

Living Independently and Home Health Care
Most seniors and many people with COPD who own their own homes want to stay there. Home health care is covered by Medicare, Medicaid

and most health insurances. They are administered a bit differently in each state, so the list of services might vary, but home health care can include nursing, home health aides, physical therapists, and occupational, respiratory, and speech therapists. Ask your doctor if you quality for home health care, and see www.eldercare.gov or call 1-800-677-1116. You can also look up Medicare certified agencies in your area and the services covered by visiting www.medicare.gov and look for the link to home health care agencies in your area, or you can call 1-800-Medicare. Local home health care agencies are great sources of information on what is and what is not available in your community.

Be aware that it is also unlawful for anyone to discriminate against you in housing. This includes private housing. If you rent, for example, your landlord is required to allow you to make reasonable accommodations to your rental space (because of the Americans with Disability Act). However, the changes must be completed at your own expense and you have to agree with the landlord to restore the property to its original condition when you leave.

ADA Information Line
(800) 514-0301 (voice)
(800) 514-0383 (TTY)
www.ada.gov

Sometimes, the barrier to remaining in one's own home is economic. Reverse mortgages were created by HUD (U.S. Department of Housing and Urban Development) and are federally insured private loans based on converting part of the equity in your home into cash. The loan provides income and is not repayable until the home is no longer your primary residence. For more information, contact AARP, 1-800-209-8085, or:

U.S. Department of Housing and Urban Development
451 7th Street SW
Washington, DC 20410
Telephone: (202) 708-1112 TTY: (202) 708-1455

Living with Family Members

If living on your own even with home care or home health care is not possible, you might want to consider moving in with a family member.

Before you consider living with a family member, be sure you read the chapter called "Families of People with COPD."

Roommates

There is no reason why people can't find others in need of help like themselves and share the expenses. This type of arrangement is very much a business arrangement, and everything should be in writing.

Co-op Housing Communities

These are a rather new phenomenon and are not co-op apartments but people working together cooperatively within an urban community who, for a fee, join a cooperative from which they can purchase services for home care, handyman help, medical escorts, etc. These are rare but becoming more popular. They are sometimes referred to as "aging in place" programs.

Specialized Living Arrangements

Before we get into describing special housing, I have to warn you that there is mass confusion when it comes to their names. One type (dare I say "assisted living") supposedly is called twenty-six different things depending on the state in which the facility is located. Further, even though you may find some types of facilities that go by the same name, the services offered might vary not only from state to state but even in the same state. Consequently, don't assume anything based on the names, even the ones I am using!

Independent Living/Supportive Housing/Senior Housing

These are government-subsidized apartment complexes for seniors on limited incomes. They are usually regular apartments or something close to them. Some are private for-profit enterprises where the landlord receives money from HUD (U.S. Department of Housing and Urban Development), and some are not-for-profit apartment complexes run by nonprofit agencies. They do not provide personal care (also called, ugh, custodial care) or medical services. Some, however, provide meals, light housekeeping, shopping, laundry, social activities, and transportation. But be aware—the services vary widely!

Board and Care Homes

Some are privately run for profit and some are voluntary not-for-profit, and they provide group living arrangements as well as help with activities such as eating, bathing, eating, etc. They are not highly regulated and monitored, and usually do not receive payment from Medicare or Medicaid; however, private or long-term care insurance may help cover the costs. In some cases, monthly charges are a percentage of your income. These are often referred to as the smaller version or type of assisted living.

Assisted Living (Congregate Living, Supportive Living, Domiciliary, Sheltered Housing, etc.)

Assisted living centers vary widely in size from about twenty units to a couple of hundred units in large high-rise facilities. Accommodations can range from one room to full apartments. There are no standard blueprints for what services they provide because each state has its own regulations. They can be operated both as for-profit and not-for-profit. They can provide a range of services such as help with activities of daily living like eating, bathing, and using the bathroom, taking medicines, and getting to appointments. Some have communal meals and some do not; some offer health care service on site and others do not. Yet others provide social workers, counselors, and other professional staff and some... well, you know the drill! The cost depends on the type of facility as well as the location and services available. Considering the cost of private housing and paying for services, these can be a good deal. They are not paid for directly by Medicare; however, Medicaid may pay for them in some states. Some of them are as "top of the line" as the continuing care retirement communities described below. Two good sources for more information are the Assisted Living Federation of America, www.alfa.org or (703) 894-1805, and the National Center for Assisted Living, www.ncal.org or (202) 842-4444.

Continuing Care Retirement Community (CCRCs)

These are often considered top of the line, but there are some assisted living centers that can give CCRCs a run for their money! CCRCs are retirement communities, often complete with luxuries such as pools, spas, golf, etc., where you have your own apartment, cottage, duplex, kingdom, etc. They also have assisted living facilities and a nursing home built into their service so that they are immediately available as your needs change. Some even have their own hospital. This "continuum of care" is a very attractive arrangement for many people. They require a substantial "entrance fee" from about $40,000 to $500,000 or more (as of 2009) as well as monthly payments.

Nursing Homes (Skilled Nursing Facility)

Most of us know what nursing homes are and hope that by reading this chapter, we find a way to avoid one. Many but certainly not all residents find them a bit more comfortable than they anticipated, usually due to the other people they meet there and the companionship they offer. Some people find them more attractive after they've experienced living alone and being relatively isolated.

Nursing homes that accept Medicare and Medicaid as well as private pay are known as skilled nursing facilities. There are others around that are just called nursing facilities, and they are not paid for by Medicare; they are private pay.

One of the secrets of nursing homes is that they usually make more money on the private pay patient than the Medicaid patient (which is where most end up), so there is an incentive for them to take in people who can afford the care—the longer they can afford to be private pay, the better.

Don't wait until you need a nursing home to find one! If you need one, you are probably too sick to look around and someone else, such as the hospital, will pick one for you, often based on who has space. Visit a few nursing homes when you are able and talk, okay, gossip with the staff and residents. If you talk to them in front of the person giving you the tour, staff will lie through their teeth and everyone you see will be on his or her best behavior. Make friends with a resident and go back to talk to him or her privately.

Hospices

Hospices are programs set up for individuals who doctors believe and certify are within six months of dying. The focus of hospice care is quality of life over quantity of days left. They strive to provide dignity and comfort. The care is palliative (soothing the symptoms) instead of curing or treating the disease. Hospice services are covered by Medicare and most medical insurance policies. Hospice services can continue for longer than six months as long as the doctor in charge periodically certifies that the person is thought to be within six months of death. They are sometimes free-standing facilities with a few rooms, or a wing in a nursing home, although more commonly they are provided in one's home—as long as the person has a primary caregiver. There are not enough free-standing hospice centers. Most are fantastic, but there are a few that are poorly run.

We cannot talk about nursing homes and hospice programs without acknowledging that they, too, are only temporary living arrangements. The inevitable for all of us, with or without COPD, is death. Most of us have thought about our death, and some of us can't stop thinking about it. Being ill and probably having too much time on our hands has, no doubt, compelled many of us to reflect upon our lives, try to make sense of our experience here on earth, and think, or perhaps worry, about our ultimate departure.

Chapter 26

PUT IT IN WRITING! PAPERWORK: WILLS, ADVANCED DIRECTIVES, ETC.

There will come a time when winter will ask what you were doing all summer.
~ Henry Clay

The hardest part of planning for the future is accepting the need to think ahead and to make important decisions now, even if you feel somewhat unprepared to make some of the big decisions. Once you get over that first hurdle of recognizing the need to make some of the harder decisions, you then have to be sure they will be honored; this requires not only putting them in writing but also doing it in a manner that is in accordance with your state's laws. The laws in each state vary, although many states recognize each other's laws under the policy of "full faith and credit" regarding health care directives and wills. It is, nevertheless, still safer to think of the paperwork as state specific unless your legal advisor informs you otherwise.

Many of us would like to postpone having to deal with the arduous task of facing our medical vulnerabilities, mortality, and last wishes. Somehow, completing one's will and medical directives is often experienced as signaling a turning point, or even a type of announcement to ourselves and others that we see the end of our life looming on the horizon. Frequently, when initiating this paperwork, we might even be asked if we are withholding information about our health or if we anticipate dying soon, so be prepared with a witty comeback if asked! Sometimes we postpone this task because we do not feel ready to make some decisions we know will be required in order to complete the paperwork; we tell ourselves we'll get to the paperwork after we've "made up our minds." Rather than knowing what you want and then putting the paperwork together, it can work the opposite way—consulting an attorney and discussing the paperwork can stimulate your thinking and help you make decisions, so don't worry about not feeling fully ready. Attorneys who specialize in estate planning are experienced and well-prepared to help you make decisions by laying out your options along with positives and negatives of each.

Not surprisingly, our values often change as we get older and we face new situations we could only once imagine. When we face those new situations, we may rethink some of our beliefs and want to change our written directives accordingly. If you understand and accept that you are allowed to rethink things and can make amendments to your directives, it makes the task a bit easier to face. What is important to know is that once the paperwork is completed, you can, for the most part, change your mind and redo what you desire. When doing any planning, make sure you discuss the possibilities of future changes with your attorney to find out for sure if your decisions are indeed revocable, and how you would go about amending them.

We are frequently reluctant to complete our paperwork because it not only requires we face the inevitability of our own death, it also may necessitate that we consider some gory medical details and worst-case scenarios. In fact, not planning for worst-case scenarios is not adequate planning. Imagining our final days or even considering the fact many of us will be "too out of it" to make our own decisions is very anxiety provoking. Yet it is easier to "bite the bullet" and get these things done now so we don't have to worry about them in the future. Oddly enough, as we struggle to maintain control over our lives due to the ravages of COPD, we shy away from this one area in which we have control. The consequences of not taking control can be great, and the benefits of taking control can be many. Regardless of our health or even the degree to which our COPD affects our lives, it is wise for all adults to get their formal paperwork completed. Although we can become almost exclusively focused on our COPD, other things can happen. Hey, you could have a heart attack when you realize you finally won the lottery!

Still want to procrastinate a bit? Well, here's another reason not to: in addition to being in your own best interest to get this chore out of the way, it is also the fair thing to do for your family. No one should have to "get stuck" making decisions on your behalf or have to try to imagine what you would want, or rely, for example, on some side comment you made about life-support after watching a dramatic and tearful made-for-TV movie! Not being prepared might also result in unnecessary legal expenses and wasted important time. Most important is that if you do what you need to do now, you might spare loved ones a great deal of emotional pain. Frankly, the whole thing is not that hard and probably not as expensive as you anticipate either. The hardest step is, of course, the first step—setting up an appointment with an attorney. So just do it.

The biggest technical problem is that not all states handle this paperwork the same, so you are going to have to check on your state laws regarding what is required. The safest way to do this is by getting a local attorney to put the paperwork together for you. After believing for twelve years that I had all my paperwork properly completed because I used a popular computer program for all the paperwork they said was specific to my state, I found out years later that the paperwork was inadequate and might not have held up in court. Even if it was eventually upheld, it would probably have required extra legal fees to ensure my meager estate went where I wanted. What I found most useful when eventually putting my papers together correctly with an attorney was the unexpected little pointers or tips she offered that I did not, or would not, have considered. Those tips were as valuable as the paperwork itself, and it was well worth the fee. Knowing my paperwork was completed correctly reassures me things will go as I plan and want. This is comforting, very comforting.

Because state laws vary, if you decide to move at any point, or if the townspeople gather once again to chase you over the state line, double check to be sure your paperwork complies with your new state's laws.

As we have encountered in other discussions, there are too many terms floating around which can make things appear more complicated than they really are. Some things go by more than one name or vary state to state. Be aware that the following is a general overview and may not accurately reflect either the terminology or the laws of your particular state. Bottom line and regardless of terms used, you want to ensure:

- your medical care is the type of care you have chosen even when you are not able to make choices or advocate for yourself;

- you have someone you trust to make medical decisions on your behalf when you are unable to make them;

- you have the power to decide beforehand what life support you want and do not want when it is unlikely you will regain consciousness;

- you have someone you trust to have the authority to take care of your nonmedical business, including financial interests, while you are alive and are unable to do so for yourself;

- upon your death, your estate will be handled and distributed according to your wishes;

- your remains are handled according to your wishes.

Advanced Directives

Advanced directives are written instructions that specify what health care you want or do not want if you are sick or injured. You can make your decisions regarding care and treatment choices now (in writing) and/or name someone to make those decisions for you (see "Health Care Power of Attorney" below). Advanced directives not only tell health professionals what you want and do not want, they also make your wishes clear to family members. Family members shouldn't have to guess or even argue about what you would want. Directives are a must. Nursing homes and hospitals usually inform you of advanced directives and can often assist you. A surprising number of people never actually sit down and discuss their desires with family members; don't be one of them! Don't just complete the forms and think your work is over—oh no! Sit down and discuss your desires with your family. It is better to make it a bit formal, perhaps having coffee at the kitchen table with the expressed purpose of talking about your desires, rather than to try to pass this important information on in dribs and drabs. Blurting out what you want or do not want while shopping or watching TV doesn't cut it!

Living Will

A living will is a formal document that provides instructions, but is different from other advanced directives in that it deals with the issue of life support when you are deemed to be in a terminal condition by your doctor and are not able to speak for yourself. (The advanced directive will address care before you get to that stage, i.e., if you are unconscious but not terminal). In your living will, you can identify what life supports—such as CPR (cardiopulmonary resuscitation), blood transfusions, feeding tubes, water, or the use of ventilators—you want and do not want.

There is a registry available that keeps your living will information for you as well as provides important and useful information about living wills. It can be found at www.uslivingwillregistry.com.

DNR Orders (Do Not Resuscitate)

Yes, we are already becoming redundant. I warned you! Some people don't get to the other more detailed advanced directives described above and just focus on one of the big ones, the DNR (do not resuscitate) order. Hospitals also push this. If you need to be resuscitated (revived from unconsciousness or possible impending death), it is something that has to be done immediately, and medical personnel do not have time to start asking questions. Medical providers need to know what to do if you stop breathing or your heart stops. Unless you have a DNR order, you will be revived. A DNR order covers this one aspect of intervention, and the forms are often provided by the hospital. Please be advised, however, that a DNR instructs the medical personnel to not attempt to resuscitate you even though there may be a chance of full recovery with this intervention. Hospitals and doctors lose them, so you may need to complete a new one each time you are admitted to a hospital, need to carry one with you, etc. DNR orders can also be part of your living will.

Organ Donation

You can decide now if you want your organs donated to others or your body to science. You can decide on one or the other or both, because people sometimes have specific preferences. It is handled differently in different states, and donation opportunities are sometimes done right along with your driver's license. Organ donation cards are often carried in one's wallet. You can learn more by calling (888) ASK-HRSA or visiting www.organdonor.com.

Power of Attorney

A power of attorney authorizes someone you designate to make decisions for you. There are different types:

- Health Care Power of Attorney (also known as Health Care Proxy): This allows an appointed individual to make medical decisions when you are not able to do so yourself as determined by your physician. How this works depends upon the laws of your particular state. You can specify the types of decisions they can make and impose any limits that you want—if you complete the required paperwork, of course. The proxy is no longer in effect when you are once again able to make your own decisions regarding your care. Be sure your doctor has a copy in your medical records, as well as the person named as your representative. Do not confuse the health care power of attorney with the financial power of attorney; they are different. Although the health care proxy applies only to your health care decisions, it is not uncommon for the same person to be named both the financial power of attorney and health care power of attorney; the choice is yours. Once again, the health care power of attorney (or health care proxy) is different from the living will. The health care power of attorney can make medical decision when you are unable, but the living will takes it a step further and specifies exactly what life support you want or do not want when it is unlikely you will recover or benefit from further treatment.

- Financial power of attorney: This gives a designated person the power or authorization to handle your nonmedical affairs, such as property and finances. Shy away from naming a shopaholic as your financial power of attorney!

Types of Power of Attorney

When you appoint someone as your power of attorney (either medical or financial or both), you have a choice of granting them one of three types of power:

- Durable power of attorney: This gives your appointed agent legal authority (limited or other) to handle your affairs. It takes effect immediately and remains valid until you either revoke it or die. It remains in effect even if you can no longer make decisions for yourself. Some people mistakenly believe your power of attorney agent can handle your affairs after you die, but he or she cannot. The power ends with your death.

- Springing power of attorney: This is the same as the durable power of attorney except that it only becomes effective when you are incapacitated as determined by a medical professional.

- Nondurable power of attorney: This is often done for limited or specific transactions. The big difference is that your designee's power continues either until you revoke it or you become unable to make your own decisions. If you are unable to make decisions, your designee is legally not allowed to act on your behalf.

It is important to know that no one watches over the power-of-attorney agents. They are on their own and report to no one but you. You can name more than one person as power of attorney if you desire.

Discuss Your Plans
You might also want to discuss your plans with your physician prior to formalizing them; your doctor might bring up some interesting points you ordinarily might not consider and answer any questions you might have. Because doctors have a huge patient load, it is not reasonable to assume they will remember the finer details of your discussions or even be able to locate copies of the paperwork you gave him or her. In the event it is needed, your doctor will most likely turn to your next of kin for assistance in locating any required documentation.

Make Copies
Be sure to make many copies of all of your paperwork and to include a copy that is kept in a safe place. Give copies to those named in the documents involved in your care, and keep copies on hand to take to your doctor and hospital. As it is with doctors, don't assume your hospital will keep important papers on file or even find them after they promise to store them. Make plenty of copies so you or your representative/advocate can grab one when needed.

Ventilators for Us COPDers
One of the hardest decisions that people need to make is whether to be put on a breathing machine—a ventilator. It may also be referred to as "being intubated," which simply means inserting a tube to aid breathing which is then hooked up to a ventilator machine. At times, a ventilator might be referred to as a "respirator," which, although technically different from a ventilator, is a term often used interchangeably in common lingo. Most medical staff have given up trying to

correct us or explain the difference. A large number of people immediately think of being put on a ventilator as something negative—something that only prolongs an unsatisfactory existence. There has been sporadic media hype and interesting lawsuits that may not always accurately reflect the situations most of us will face. A ventilator is a piece of life-support equipment, and there is a big difference between being put on life support when there is only the slimmest chance of survival and being put on life support on a temporary basis as part of active medical treatment. Because we have a lung disease, we need to perhaps approach the discussion of whether to be intubated (put on a ventilator) a bit differently than most people. Because of our COPD, we may need to be on a ventilator when fighting an infection or other disease, or simply to compensate for our lousy lungs when recovering from an illness or surgery. Our chance of needing a ventilator during an illness (particularly one that affects the lungs) is greater than average. Be absolutely sure that you, your family, and your health care proxy understand the difference between using a ventilator as a support through an illness and being on a ventilator when there is little, if any, chance of recovery. As a matter of fact, if you need to put this book down right now to tell them, I will understand! If needed, you'll find a longer discussion of ventilators in the chapter on hospitalizations. I know a number of people who are still around and having a good time who have been on ventilators when they were critically ill; in almost all cases they were unable to make the decision on their own at the time. If they hadn't allowed a ventilator, they would clearly have made a big mistake. This is also when a DNR order can be counterproductive. If need be, please discuss DNR orders or any concerns you have regarding the use of a ventilator with your doctor. If once on a ventilator you cannot be wean off of one, your living will is there to protect you.

Last Will and Testament
We all know what a will is, and many of us have one, often outdated! Review your will to ensure it is up to date and my name is spelled correctly!

People tend to be more prepared to complete their will than they are the health care paperwork, probably because they have strong feelings about who should or should not have their belongings when they die. It is, indeed, your last statement. Some people even make a video recording to let their family and friends hear their final thoughts and to communicate with family members unborn or too young to remember them. If you plan on leaving a video statement, check with your attorney to be sure it will not compromise your last will and testament.

Because anyone can contest a will (which will hold up the process), it is important that it be constructed with that in mind. An attorney has ways to decrease the chances that it will be contested. Mine came up with some very valuable tips. You do not want your estate stuck with legal bills because you failed to complete your will in the best way possible.

Remember you can change your will at any time as long as you are competent. Of course, we all know the stories of people challenging wills because they were made under duress or when the person was incompetent (or so it was claimed). Whether you share the contents of your will with anyone is your business. You may choose, like me, to tell everyone but the mailman they are your sole beneficiary and that you will definitely change your will if they mention it to anyone. It not only keeps them silent, but they also send better quality chocolates when I'm sick. I'm sure my attorney would advise me against this amusing practice for fear my dubious actions might later be used to prove my insanity!

As tempting as it is to manipulate people by talking about your will (or lying about it), if you do just happen to bring it up in conversation, you then have to wonder if they are being kind or unkind to you because of what you say. Yes, fear of being taken out of your will or promises to be put in can motivate people, but you need to be aware the manipulation is often resented. Most of us have seen people try to control others through making statements (often promises or threats) about their will, but few of us have ever seen any good ever come from it. Perhaps the best approach is to keep them guessing and to share little, if any, information about the contents of your will. However, this is a personal matter and one for you to discuss with your attorney.

If you have a designated power of attorney, be aware that person's power ends upon your death. The person who will oversee the distribution of your estate is the executor named in your will. Your will must be submitted to probate (surrogates) court to prove the validity of your will. Your executor will oversee the process and protect the estate. Once your will is admitted to probate, your executor will distribute the assets according to your written wishes. The time frame is particular to each case. Your executor should know to contact your attorney upon your death, or shortly thereafter, to discuss mutual responsibilities. An executor does not have to deal with the finer details of distributing your estate; he or she can retain an attorney to assist in the process and to take care of the work involved. An executor is entitled to commissions to administer your estate.

There are some assets that bypass the will, such as life insurance policies, joint bank and other accounts, or other assets that are "payable upon death." Although they may still be taxed, they go directly to the individual named. This is part of the estate planning you should discuss with your attorney. Rather than just think about your last will and testament, you might want to broaden your options and discuss "estate planning" with your attorney. In estate planning, there are often major advantages of setting things up sooner rather than later, especially if there is any chance that one might need to rely one day on public assistance.

You should also discuss "living trusts" with your attorney. These are estate planning documents that are set up to bypass your will and avoid probate, often saving money in the process. The laws, fees, taxes, and other considerations particular to your estate should once again, you guessed it, be discussed with your attorney.

If you die without a will, your estate still may need to go to surrogates court. In some states your assets go directly to your spouse. In some states the will still needs to go through surrogates and an administrator will be named by the court. The property distribution is then in accordance to state law, not your wishes. It is all rather complex and explains why you need to do proper estate planning with your attorney.

Funeral Arrangements

There are three ways you can deal with your funeral and burial.

1. Leave it to your agent to take care of.

2. Plan your funeral and burial by identifying in writing specifically what you want and leaving it for your executor to handle pursuant to written instructions.

3. Plan your funeral and burial and enter an agreement with a funeral home.

Let's face it, no one wants to have to make funeral arrangements either for themselves or someone else, but someone has to do it. One thing is clear: it is very hard to make funeral arrangements when you are in shock or mourning someone's death. Frankly, leaving your arrangements to someone else is a lot to expect of loved ones—although a good argument can be made that the ritual of going to a funeral home and making the arrangements helps the grieving process. The person making the arrangements is at a disadvantage if he or she equates the expense of the arrangement with the expression of love and grief.

You can make funeral arrangements ahead of time with a funeral home so that everything is set upon your death. Not everyone has the disposition to do this, and if you can't, that's okay. You can only do what you can do. If you do make arrangements, the details of the arrangement can be left with your executor, who can contact the funeral home upon your death, therefore sparing others the task of planning your funeral.

Prearranging your funeral is entering an agreement or legal contract with the funeral home, so you must be careful. If you enter an agreement with the funeral home, are the prices guaranteed? What happens if, due to inflation, prices go up? Your funeral home will be concerned with where the money is coming from to pay for your funeral. Be safe, consider this right along with your estate planning, and get your attorney's advice.

You can also prepay your funeral. How this works and the laws governing this, once again, depend on your state. Is the price you are paying guaranteed to remain in effect until your death? Does the money you've prepaid earn interest? If so, what happens to the interest? Is it kept to offset the costs that go up due to inflation? What happens if the funeral home closes or is sold? What if you want to change your plans or want your money back? What if you move out of the area? One commonly mentioned advantage is that you can make arrangements and pay today's prices. The reverse of the argument is that you could invest that same amount of money, accrue the interest and still be ahead after paying the costs that increase over the years.

Those who advocate investing the money tend to forget you will not be around to spend the interest!

Also, if you are on public assistance of any sort, including Medicaid or Supplemental Social Security, find out if your state allows you to set aside money for burial expenses and, if so, how much it allows. Ordinarily, if you have prepaid funeral plans that were paid for before you applied for public assistance, the state may not be able to take it away although it may have an issue with the amount you paid and insist the plans be modified accordingly. Check this all out before you make plans.

Regardless of your plans, be they general guidelines, a specific detailed request, or an agreement (prepaid or not with a funeral home), be sure to let people know about it, and keep a copy of the arrangements in the location you keep your important papers.

Be aware that you can legally appoint someone to be the agent to control the disposition of your remains. Speak to your attorney about this.

Other Paperwork

It is advisable to create a file where other important papers are located. Be sure to tell chosen individuals where the file is kept! Within the file, keep all the information they would need regarding safe deposit boxes, income, financial institutions with whom you have relationships, marriage licenses, military papers, insurance information, deeds, ownership papers, funeral arrangements (if any), and phone numbers of people to contact if you die. I have assured my executors they will find everything they need in this file and they know where it is kept. Having brought it up, I really should update it! A good time to check and update your file is at tax time, as you will no doubt already be sad and tearful.

Beyond Paperwork

You can have all the paperwork completed, witnessed, crossed all the "t's" and dotted all the "i's" but that is only one part of being prepared for the inevitable. The inevitable for all of us, with and without COPD, is death. Most of us have thought about it, and some of us can't stop thinking about it. There are things you can do to come to terms with death and dying, and perhaps even ease some of the fears many of us have.

Chapter 27

DEATH AND DYING: THE FINAL FRONTIER

Death is not the greatest loss in life. The greatest loss is what dies inside us while we live.
~Norman Cousins

Death and Dying

We've come a long way together. We first started out talking about being diagnosed with COPD and how to break the news to family and friends, and here we are now, talking about death and dying—perhaps not an uplifting subject to end a book, but fitting nonetheless. Coming to terms with the inevitability of death, be it our own or others, is perhaps one of the hardest challenges of our lives. However, accepting the inevitability of our own death may actually allow us to focus more on living. Truly accepting death usually requires that we also make sense of our lives. Coming to terms with our life and death can be as much an act of appreciation and subdued celebration as it is a preparation for a sad farewell.

Most people are more afraid of *how* they die rather than death itself. This holds especially true for people with COPD, because we are often afraid of suffocating to death and of leaving this earth gasping and terrified. The first thing we need to do is dispense with this gruesome expectation. It certainly is understandable why many of us have this terrifying image and why we are afraid of dying; however, it is an inaccurate image. Frankly, our passing is almost always much less dramatic—we are medicated, relatively pain free, and less attuned to what is going on around us than we imagine. Any discomfort we experience is prior to getting to a hospital or being on hospice. Morphine, I've been assured, eases the sensation of shortness of breath and makes one comfortable. No one can promise you a comfortable passing, but it appears the anticipation is much worse than the experience itself.

Coming to terms with our death is also about coming to terms with our lives. So much of our concern and distress with having COPD lies in how it robs us of some of the physical opportunities that life offers. We also know that although it does change the list of things we are able to do, it does not have to change the level of enjoyment of those things we are still able to do. Happiness and joy come from within, not from outside of us. A beautiful sunset is not in and of itself joyful; the sun is a fireball devoid of feelings. Our reaction to it, joy or awe, is what makes it beautiful. Colorful fall leaves do not embody amazement; amazement is our reaction to the array of colors. The appreciation comes from within us, not from within the trees. Some of us stare in awe at the beauty of the leaves, and others take them for granted. Still others mumble obscenities at the thought of having to rake them. Yet others of us don't even need the real thing; we can appreciate nature's display through pictures, and we can even imagine the smell of the musty fall earth when we gaze at the array of colorful fall leaves in a picture. Similarly, although goodbyes will always be sad, death and dying is what we make of it. It does not have to be about suffering, fear, and grief.

In addition to physical suffering, most of us also fear the emotional suffering that may precede and accompany our deaths. I once attended a group led by an experienced and rather wise and mature nun with many years of experience working with terminally ill people. She was asked by one young man who was terminally ill to describe what dying was like. You could see the fear, almost terror on his face. Her response was simple. She explained in a calm and reassuring voice that everyone she has been with who has died, which were many, experienced death in the same way they experienced life—how they lived was how they died, and it was no more complicated than that. If you've been miserable throughout your life, your death will be no different, and if you embraced life and lived a dignified life, you will die with love and dignity. She further explained that dying is part of our life and we depart in the same style we lived—we don't change at the end. Death is, like everything else in life, what you make of it. Being healthy at the time I heard her speak, I realized you don't have to be near your own death in order to accept it. We can all benefit, no doubt, healthy or ill, by coming to terms with death and dying; it is too profound and valuable to squander on the frail and elderly.

Coming to terms with the inevitable end of our lives is one of the most important gifts we can give ourselves.

Thus far we have learned about holding onto life and taking as much control over our disease as possible. We have learned about our disease and figured out how to get the best medical care we can. We tried to face the emotional problems that often accompany COPD and even looked upon the impact our illness has upon our family and friends. We tried to harness the COPD beast by taking control of our illness right down to understanding the paperwork that will ensure we will be treated in the manner we desire. It is now time to flip the coin over and take a look at the other side—the benefits of accepting that our time, like everyone's, is limited and that there are some things we can't control. We've learned to hold on to those things that are important to us, but there is also a time to let go of those things that hold us back. For many of us, letting go is harder than holding on.

Some of us will struggle more than others with the idea of departing this world, and much of it has to do with concern for the well-being of those we leave behind. Although we're all in the same boat, it is very hard for many of us to accept and deal with death, and if you are having a very difficult time of it, it is understandable. The amount of struggle, perhaps, foreshadows the magnitude of the reward. Unlike us, some people depart suddenly and don't have the opportunity to reflect upon and accept their own mortality. Others who we have known and loved simply refuse to accept the reality of their mortality—much like indestructible perpetual teenagers. Still others accept their mortality, prepare as best they can, and wait out their days, watching the clock and feeling life is over. However, even in our most difficult moments, we need to remind ourselves that life isn't over until it's over. Until we let go of life, we can still take advantage of being alive. Accepting and coming to terms with our death allows us to assuage our fear of death, frees us up, and let us get back to living and enjoying what time we do have. It is hard to enjoy life if we live in fear of dying.

Life, like Shakespeare said, is a stage and we are all but actors. Ideally, we need to accept that our time on this stage will one day be over and, if need be, we should be prepared to provide our own applause if the theatre is empty. We can complain about our poor health, but we do not have to be in good health to be happy. Being happy can be our way of expressing our rage and indignation against COPD; there is no better revenge—kind of like praying in front of the devil just to annoy him.

I'm not pretending that coming to terms with our own death is easy; it is far from it, but it can be done. Accepting and coming to terms with one's own life and inevitable death can allow an intensity to life we can only recall from early childhood days, before we "grew up." It is possible, even now, to start living life more fully. People who know their days are numbered often report waking up from a stupor; they report having clarity of mind greater than they've ever experienced. They "let go" of the things that get in the way of living so that they can grab onto and savor those things that really matter. They focus not on the past or the future, but on the moment. They squeeze as much life from each moment as possible. They become more alive, more appreciative of every day they have, and live with their senses heighten. Their only regret is that they didn't discover this way of being earlier. Yes, they continue to have hard days, they continue to experience sadness and even suffering, but even those painful moments have new meaning. No, their heads are not in the clouds, they are above them. If they can soar above the clouds, so can each one of us. We can have rich lives regardless of our COPD and find meaning in our lives and our deaths. We can die with dignity and leave this world a better place for having had us as a guest. COPD can't rob us of that unless we let it.

More than anything, coming to terms with death is often a direct challenge to our beliefs. Sometimes things need to unravel before they can be reconstructed. Dealing with our death requires we confront our own fears and expectations about death and the afterlife. It is an opportunity to examine our beliefs, amend, or even radically change them. We are wiser now than ever. As we approach some unknowns, some of us will discover real faith for the first time. Others will confirm their faith and, yes, a few of us, no doubt, will even lose our faith—some temporarily and some permanently. How we live is how we die. Although none of this is easy, the failure to come to terms with our lives and the end of our lives is a lost opportunity.

When we start thinking seriously about coming to the end of our lives, when we believe we only have a few months or a few years to live, it is natural for many of us to want to review our lives. We want to recall our past and replay our lives. We want to stitch all the fragments together now that we have a more complete picture of what our life is about. We hold on to memories as we do dear companions, and in doing so we keep our past and our past relationships with people we love (and hate) with us. They are alive in our memories. We perhaps wonder if, when we die, our memories will continue or if all memory will cease. Whether or not memories (or relationships) survive beyond death is a matter of individual belief along with a large dose of faith. You have the opportunity to answer this question for yourself. Reviewing one's life allows for a sense of continuity in our current lives, makes sense of the present, and reminds us we are on a journey and heading towards either our life's destination or a stopping-off point. What you believe about purpose and destination depends on your personal philosophy or religious beliefs. Those beliefs will influence, if not dictate, how you come to terms with your life and your death. Not knowing what to believe is disconcerting but useful. Contemplating the meaning of your life gives you the opportunity to explore your beliefs as well as your fears so you can finally put the matter to rest. Once completed, you can get back to living and enjoying what you have.

When reviewing our life, we will often find ourselves full of judgments regarding the past actions of others. We must either acknowledge our thankfulness if they added value to our lives or forgive them if they devalued us. Forgiving others allows us to let go of them; not forgiving others weighs down our spirit. Why? Because we are the ones with the residual bad feeling and they probably couldn't care less! If we had the opportunity to thoroughly examine the fine details of the lives of some of the creeps we've encountered or people who have harmed us, we would, more likely than not, understand why they turned out the way they did. We have all met people who are damaged. Heck, we might even consider ourselves damaged! It is easier to assume they, like us, acted the way they did for reasons beyond our knowledge. If we adopt this attitude, we can dismiss our case against them. Try to empty your courtroom while you are still on the bench. Have you ever considered that perhaps even the louts we encountered during our lives were put there for a reason? Did we learn something from having come upon them? Regardless, let the memory of them walk away and depart forever. Say goodbye to any of your ill will towards them, because the anger and hatred is certainly not doing you any good. Visualize them in your mind, tell them what you want to say, but say goodbye to them. Imagine either yourself or them comfortably walking away. Remember, we react to things in our imagination in much the same way we do to things in reality, so even this mental exercise is important. Through our ability to imagine, we can let go of the resentment and anger we've stowed away—it is unnecessary and heavy baggage. So even though it might sound corny, it does work.

Perhaps the hardest part of reviewing one's life is dealing with the report card we seem to want to complete on ourselves. To some extent, some of us have become the report card and lost touch with the person being evaluated. How did we do in love? What is our score for parenting? Did we fail the positive attitude test? Have we harmed others? We all have one thing in common: We have all been raised in an atmosphere of comparisons and evaluations. We heard we were doing a "good job" or did a "no-no" long before we even understood the true meaning of those words, and we equated those evaluations with a smile or a grimace, with love or rejection. We've had a life of being evaluated, and we learned early in our lives to be highly attuned to evaluations and to even evaluate ourselves. We gave and continue to give ourselves scores for our ability to amass material possessions, our reputation, status, education, job, etc. Frankly, although some of those things might help our physical comfort (e.g., affording a top-of-the-line mattress and private care), they are of little value in the final analysis. We are all the same once we decide to tear up the report cards. Who you are underneath those evaluations is greater and more important than any evaluation you've ever received. We are really the board upon which evaluations are tacked. The evaluations we've gotten often become so numerous and dense they obscure even the existence of the board underneath. We are not the evaluations; we are the board onto which they are tacked. We have the opportunity to remove, examine, and rearrange any and all of the evaluations, or if we can, toss them all aside.

As we review the evaluations, we might realize that many of them are related to superficial things, things we will one day leave behind.

They are like decorations on the board, attractive but not really essential. It is time to redecorate. We are not just about our success—we are about what we have learned from our failures and what we have overcome. Do not judge yourself harshly when you examine your life; forgive yourself for those things you were not prepared to be successful at. Do not live in or leave a world where you are nothing more than what you accomplished or accumulated. Get in touch with the small kid you used to be, long before you were judged and long before you got to know yourself only through your accomplishments. Live with the satisfaction that you did your best, and remember that your own applause, next to God's, is the most important applause when it is time to leave the stage.

End

INDEX

CPSIA information can be obtained at www.ICGtesting.com

227781LV00010B/19/P